Cardiovascular Risk Management

T0188378

Commissioning Editor: *Mary Banks*
Development Editor: *Kate Newell*

Cardiovascular Risk Management

Edited by

FD Richard Hobbs
The University of Birmingham
The Medical School
Birmingham B15 2TA
United Kingdom

Bruce Arroll
Professor and Head of Department of General
Practice and Primary Health Care
University of Auckland
Auckland, New Zealand

WILEY-BLACKWELL

Library of Congress Cataloging-in-Publication Data
Cardiovascular risk management/edited by Richard Hobbs, Bruce Arroll.
    p. ; cm.
  Includes bibliographical references and index.
  ISBN 978-1-4051-5575-5 (pbk. : alk. paper)
  1. Cardiovascular system—Diseases—Risk factors.   2. Cardiovascular system—Diseases—prevention.
I. Hobbs, Richard, M.R.C.G.P.   II. Arroll, Bruce.
  [DNLM: 1. Cardiovascular Diseases—prevention & control.   2. Risk Assessment. WG 120 C26778 2008]

RC682.C43 2008
616.1—dc22   2008026350

A catalogue record for this book is available from the British Library.

Set in 9.5/12 Times New Roman by Charon Tec Ltd (A Macmillan Company) www.macmillansolutions.com

Printed & bound in Singapore by Fabulous Printers Pte Ltd

1   2008

Contents

Foreword

Cardiovascular disease (CVD) has become a global health challenge. The traditional medical paradigm of assessing and treating single risk factors – hypertension, hypercholesterolemia and hyperglycaemia – as isolated diseases has been replaced by the concept of total cardiovascular risk assessment and management, as advocated by the World Health Organisation and other guidance on CVD prevention. Clinicians are now expected to ask the question 'What is my patients total risk of developing CVD?' namely the probability of developing symptomatic CVD over a defined time period, through integration of all available information on their cardiovascular risk factors. Those at highest total CVD risk can then be medically targeted, initially by lifestyle, and then the appropriate use of cardioprotective medications, in order to reduce their total CVD risk. This short book on cardiovascular risk management summarises the current clinical guidelines on CVD prevention, the different approaches to assessing total CVD risk in our patients, and how to comprehensively manage that risk. It reinforces the new medical paradigm of total risk assessment and management and provides clinicians with contemporary guidance on the primacy of professional lifestyle interventions and therapeutic management of blood pressure, lipids and glucose. Clinicians have an important responsibility to identify those patients in their practice who, because they are at high CVD risk, will gain most benefit from a preventive cardiology programme. All members of the multidisciplinary team – doctors, nurses, dieticians, physiotherapists and others – have a role in the practice of preventive cardiology. This book will help all health professionals to achieve a higher standard of care for their patients. The challenge is to do so in our every day clinical practice.

Professor David A Wood
Garfield Weston Professor of Cardiovascular Medicine
National Heart and Lung Institute
Imperial College
London UK

Contributors

B. Arroll
Professor and Head of Department of General
Practice and Primary Health Care
University of Auckland
Auckland, New Zealand

J. Betteridge
Department of Medicine, University College London
London, UK

S.A. Brunton
Cabarrus Family Medicine Residency, Charlotte,
North Carolina, USA

M.R. Cowie
Professor of Cardiology,
National Heart & Lung Institute Imperial College
London, UK

D. Duhot
General Practitioner
Société Française de Médecine Générale
Issy les Moulineaux, France

L. Erhardt
Professor of Cardiology
Department of Cardiology Malmö University Hospital
Malmö, Sweden

C.R. Elley
University of Auckland, Auckland,
New Zealand

A. Fitton
Senior Editor
The Future Forum Secretariat
London, UK

F.D.R. Hobbs
Professor and Head of Primary Care and General Practice
Primary Care Clinical Sciences Building
University of Birmingham
Birmingham, UK

A.W. Hoes
Professor of Clinical Epidemiology and General Practice
Julius Center for Health Sciences and Primary Care
University Medical
Center Utrecht
Utrecht, The Netherlands

R. Jackson
Professor of Epidemiology
Head of Epidemiology & Biostatistics
School of Population Health
Tamaki Campus
University of Auckland,
Auckland, New Zealand

T. Kenealy
Associate Professor of Integrated care,
Department of General Practice and
Primary Health Care,
University of Auckland,
Auckland, New Zealand

L.A. Leiter
Professor of Medicine and Nutrition Sciences,
University of Toronto,
Toronto, Canada

H. Lebovitz
State University of New York
Health Science Center,
New York, NY, USA

S. Mann
Department of Medicine
University of Otago
Wellington Clinical School
Wellington, New Zealand

E. McGregor
Senior Editor
The Future Forum Secretariat
London, UK

J. Mendive

Family Physician
La MZina Health Centre
Catalan Health Institute
Barcelona, Spain

A.G. Olsson

Faculty of Health Sciences,
Linköping University, Sweden

C. Packard

Department of Pathological Biochemistry
Glasgow Royal Infirmary
Alexandra Parade
Glasgow, UK

F. Sacks

Professor of Cardiovascular Disease Prevention
Nutrition Department
Harvard School of Public Health;
Professor of Medicine
Cardiovascular Division and Channing Laboratory
Brigham & Women's Hospital
Harvard Medical School
Boston, USA

J. Shepherd

Department of Vascular Biochemistry
Division of Cardiovascular and Medical Sciences
Glasgow Royal Infirmary
North Glasgow University Hospital Division
Glasgow, UK

J.I. Stewart

Lecturer, Rural Family Practice, University of Toronto
Toronto, Canada

A. Tonkin

Department of Epidemiology and Preventive Medicine
Monash University
Melbourne, Australia

E. Washbrook

Senior Editor
The Future Forum Secretariat
London, UK

S. Wells

Senior Lecturer Clinical Epidemiology
Section of Epidemiology and Biostatistics
School of Population Health
Tamaki Campus
University of Auckland
Auckland, New Zealand

The epidemiology of cardiovascular disease

F.D.R. Hobbs[1], A.W. Hoes[2], and M.R. Cowie[3]

[1]University of Birmingham, Birmingham, UK
[2]University Medical Center Utrecht, Utrecht, The Netherlands
[3]Imperial College, London, UK

Introduction

Cardiovascular disease has become the world's major cause of death, responsible for one-third of total global deaths in 2001 and the expectation that by 2020 its continuing increase in incidence will result in it far exceeding all other causes of death and disability (Figure 1.1).[1]

Traditionally thought of as a disease of developed economies, cardiovascular mortality is now rapidly rising in developing countries, largely due to uptake of a Western lifestyle, including smoking and dietary habits. In 2001, some 80% of all cardiovascular deaths worldwide took place in developing, low- and middle-income countries, while these countries also accounted for 86% of the total global burden of cardiovascular disease.

Precise estimates of the prevalence and incidence of the major cardiovascular diseases, and of their time trends, are variably available. Existing registries, such as national mortality statistics or disease-specific hospital admission rates, do provide useful information, albeit with inherent limitations, of misclassification, changes in coding systems and lack of information on non-hospitalised patients. The initiation of long-term follow-up measurement of established population cohorts has provided insights into the occurrence of cardiovascular disease and development of cardiovascular risk factors over time. The most widely cited of these cohorts (Table 1.1)[2–11] is the Framingham Heart Study (FHS).[2]

The number of people at risk of cardiovascular disease is rising as average life expectancy increases and the economic, social and cultural changes that have led to increases in vascular risk factors continue. Of particular concern are the recent rapid rises in obesity in children and adolescents (Figure 1.2),[12] largely the result of increased caloric intake coupled

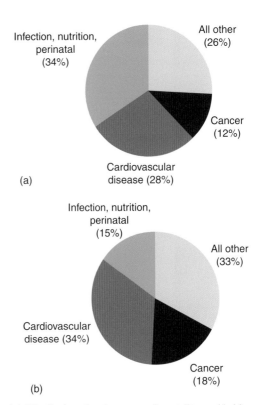

Figure 1.1 Distribution of major causes of mortality worldwide: (a) 1990 and (b) projected to 2020.[1]

with an increasingly sedentary lifestyle. This trend is predicted to increase rates of insulin resistance, which is central to a cluster of cardiovascular risk factors, and therefore add to the global burden of cardiovascular disease. Perversely, increased survival and better secondary prevention in patients suffering from cardiovascular events are further increasing prevalence of cardiovascular disease.

Although in developed countries cardiovascular disease will remain the main cause of disability and mortality, several favourable trends in the epidemic of cardiovascular disease

Cardiovascular Risk Management, Edited by R Hobbs and B Arroll
© 2009 Blackwell Publishing, ISBN: 9781405155755

Table 1.1 Examples of population-based studies that increased the knowledge in the occurrence of and determinants of cardiovascular disease

Study		Countries	Numbers	Gender	Age	Period
Framingham Heart Study[2]		USA	5,209	M/F	30–62	1948–Present
Seven Countries Study[3]		Italy, Finland, Greece, Japan, Netherlands, USA, Yugoslavia	11,579	M	40–59	1957–Present
Study of men born in 1913[4]		Sweden	792	M	54	1963–Present
Whitehall Study[5]		England	17,530	M	20–64	1967–1977
PROCAM[6]		Germany	10,856	M	36–65	1978–Present
MONICA[7]		Worldwide	10 million	M/F	25–64	1980–1995
Cardiovascular Health Study[8]		USA	5,888	M/F	65+	1989–1999
Rotterdam Study[9]		Netherlands	7,983	M/F	55+	1990–Present
INTERHEART[10,11]		Worldwide	15,152 Case 14,820 Control	M/F	No age restriction, age range not available	1999–2002

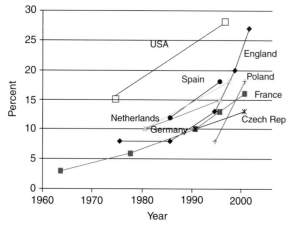

Figure 1.2 Rising prevalence of overweight children (5–11) in Europe in percentage. *Source*: Reproduced with permission from International Association for the Study of Obesity/International Obesity TaskForce.[12]

have been observed. These include a continuing decrease in the age-specific mortality rates from acute myocardial infarction (MI) since the 1970s[13] (Figure 1.3), and more recently and in fewer countries, a decrease in the number of hospitalisations

for heart failure.[14,15] The former is primarily attributable to favourable changes in modifiable risk factors (both in individuals with or without manifest vascular disease) and increased availability of mortality-reducing interventions, such as thrombolysis and interventional procedures (percutaneous transluminal coronary angioplasty), and medications for treating hypertension, hyperlipidaemia and atherothrombosis.

Improved prognosis in patients with MI, together with the ageing population and improved therapy in patients with known heart failure, is a main contributor to the sharp increase in the number of hospitalisations for heart failure observed in Western societies in the 1980s and early 1990s. More recent analyses, however, show that this growth of heart failure may have reached its peak; a decline in hospitalisation rates were documented in several countries, including Scotland[14] and the Netherlands[15] (Figure 1.4). Improved care, including pharmacotherapy, is considered the cause of this positive trend.

Risk factors for cardiovascular disease may be present in childhood or early adulthood, but it may be decades before clinical disease manifests. Therefore, early identification of patients at risk coupled with provision of optimal risk management

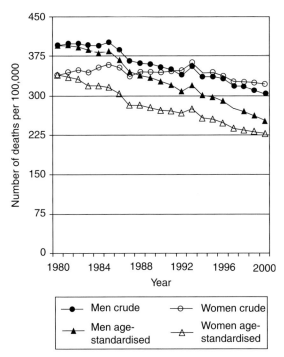

Figure 1.3 Decline in age-adjusted mortality from acute myocardial infarction in the Netherlands, 1979–2000. Mortality in 1979 was set at 100. *Source*: Reproduced with permission from statistics Netherlands. Ref. 13.

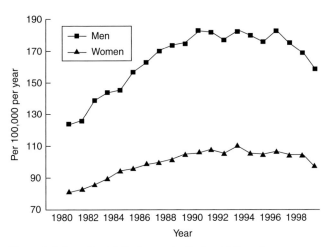

Figure 1.4 Age-adjusted discharge rates for heart failure, the Netherlands, 1980–1999. *Source*: Reproduced with permission from BMJ Publishing Group Ltd. Ref. 15.

is of vital importance in lowering the risk of cardiovascular morbidity and mortality and slowing disease progression. The reader is referred to the reference list for further background and statistics.[16–18]

Box 1.1 Classification of risk indicators

Major modifiable
- Blood pressure
- Blood lipids
- Glucose intolerance
- Cigarette smoking
- Physical activity
- Obesity
- Diet.

Non-modifiable
- Age
- Heredity or family history
- Gender
- Ethnicity
- Prior CVD.

Other modifiable
- Socioeconomic status
- Mental ill health (depression)
- Use of certain medication.

Proposed 'novel markers'
- Homocysteine levels
- Inflammatory markers (e.g. C-reactive protein)
- Blood coagulation (e.g. fibrinogen levels)
- Non-invasive measurements of atherosclerosis (e.g. carotid intima-media thickness, coronary calcifications on computerised tomography [CT] scan).

Box 1.2 Highlights of the main findings of the Framingham Heart Study[2]

- Cigarette smoking increases the risk of heart disease
- Switching to filtered cigarettes does not measurably reduce heart disease risk
- Some heart attacks are 'silent', or cause no pain
- The ratio of total cholesterol to high-density lipoprotein cholesterol (HDL-C) is a good predictor of risk
- High LDL-C leads to heart disease
- Low HDL-C leads to heart disease
- Obesity and inactivity increase the risk of heart disease
- Higher systolic or diastolic blood pressure increases the risk of heart disease

---

Risk factors for cardiovascular disease

Factors that indicate risk for coronary heart disease are well established (Box 1.1) with serum cholesterol, blood pressure and smoking identified as the three major modifiable risk factors as early as the mid-1950s.

The pivotal data came from the FHS,[2] which was initiated in 1948 to identify and evaluate factors influencing the development of cardiovascular disease in men and women free of these conditions at the outset (Box 1.2). In 1971 the Framingham Offspring study was initiated in children and spouses of the original cohort to study family patterns of cardiovascular

Box 1.3 Nine modifiable risk factors assessed in the INTERHEART study[10,11]

- Smoking
- Hypertension
- Diabetes/glucose intolerance
- Dyslipidaemia
- Obesity
- Physical activity
- Diet
- Alcohol consumption
- Psychosocial score

Box 1.4 Benefits associated with reducing blood cholesterol, blood pressure and smoking cessation

Serum cholesterol

- 10% decrease corresponds to a 30% decrease in risk of coronary heart disease.

Blood pressure

- 6 mmHg decrease in diastolic pressure > 90 mmHg (in patients with mild-to-moderate hypertension) results in a 16% decrease in coronary heart disease.

Smoking

- Cessation if cigarette smoking results in about a 50% decrease in risk of coronary heart disease.

Source: Based on data from Ref. 18.

disease and risk factors. In 2002 the Third-Generation Study began enroling grandchildren of the original enrolees.

Another important cohort of healthy men aged 40–59 years, the Seven Countries Study[3] (see Table 1.1), showed that cardiovascular risk is strongly related to both serum cholesterol and the proportion of saturated fatty acids in the diet.

Recently the INTERHEART study[10,11] confirmed that nine potentially modifiable risk factors (Box 1.3) were strongly associated with the development of a first MI by comparing patients with a first MI with asymptomatic individuals from 52 countries. The risk factors, including smoking, hypertension, diabetes, dyslipidaemia and obesity, accounted for 90% of the population risk of MI in all ethnic groups and across all geographical regions.

By the 1960s, the relationship between risk factor elevation and risk of coronary heart disease was so well established that intervention trials to determine whether reducing modifiable risk factors would reduce risk were initiated. Many studies have now established there are significant benefits to lifestyle changes and pharmacotherapy to reduce blood cholesterol, blood pressure and stop smoking (Box 1.4) both as primary prevention in at-risk individuals with no symptoms and as

secondary prevention of recurrent events in patients with established cardiovascular disease.[19]

Calculating cardiovascular risk

The wider availability of interventions that can reduce cardiovascular risk offers the potential for preventing, modifying or delaying cardiovascular disease. However, in order to treat modifiable risk factors it is necessary to identify at-risk individuals. This is simple in patients who have suffered a cardiovascular event, such as the onset of angina, since they are symptomatic. Randomised trials have shown unequivocally that risk factor intervention in these patients is cost-effective.[20] However, risk assessment in individual patients without manifest cardiovascular disease is more complex because of the need to assess the impact of multiple risk factors.

Although the population at large would certainly derive benefit from interventions aimed at primary prevention of cardiovascular disease in all individuals, such 'population strategies' are outside the scope of medicine, though there are debates over the potential of 'polypill' strategies in all middle-aged people.[21] Health systems therefore need to identify those at greatest absolute risk of cardiovascular disease to prioritise management of those with most to gain – the 'high-risk strategy'. Using such risk estimation enables health systems to nominate a risk threshold above which people are eligible for intervention, based on the ability of that society to afford treatment, by limiting the population which is at most risk to above the cut-off.

Most countries now advocate the threshold to consider initiation of pharmacological intervention to be above a 10-year risk of major cardiovascular events of 20% (or coronary heart disease of 15%). Current European guidelines advocate a 5% cardiovascular disease *mortality* threshold based on fatal, as opposed to all, cardiovascular events.[22]

Several risk calculators have been developed to better predict an individual's absolute risk of experiencing a cardiovascular event over a given period of time (e.g. 10-year risk of cardiovascular disease or coronary heart disease).[23] Currently, the most widely used risk charts and tables are based on the Framingham risk equation, using data from the FHS. Other risk algorithms have been developed, such as the Prospective Cardiovascular Munster Heart Study (PROCAM),[6,24] based on a German population. However, due to these studies being based on small populations, the risk charts have limitations (Box 1.5).

More recently, the European Systematic Coronary Risk Evaluation (SCORE) charts were created to address some of the limitations of existing risk prediction systems.[25,26] SCORE is based on asymptomatic individuals from 12 European cohort studies with no evidence of pre-existing cardiovascular disease. Studies across multiple countries enabled charts to be drawn up for high- and low-risk countries, and because atherosclerotic

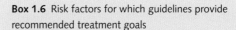

> **Box 1.5** The limitations of the Framingham study as a basis for risk calculators
>
> - Participants were mainly North American, Caucasian participants of certain socio-economic class.
> - Therefore, applicability to different ethnic and socio-economic groups is uncertain, for example, risk calculators overestimate risk in European populations.
> - Does not incorporate all risk factors.
> - Some endpoint definitions differ from those used in other studies and the choice of endpoints has changed over time.

> **Box 1.6** Risk factors for which guidelines provide recommended treatment goals
>
> - Cigarette smoking
> - Serum lipid levels
>   - LDL-C
>   - Total cholesterol
>   - Total cholesterol: HDL-C ratio
> - High blood pressure
> - Obesity/overweight
>   - Body Mass Index/waist circumference
> - Atherogenic diet
> - Physical inactivity/sedentary lifestyle.

cardiovascular disease mortality was the endpoint, these charts are expected to provide more accurate estimates of overall cardiovascular risk than algorithms predicting all cardiovascular events.

Risk calculators should be used as part of an overall strategy to identify and assess which patient is at risk and the level of treatment they require.

Guidelines for cardiovascular risk management

To effectively forestall the rising incidence of cardiovascular disease, national efforts must be made to modify lifestyle trends. To do this, strategies to reduce risk factors should be taken into account in public policy and education. In addition, identification of high-risk patients and intervention, often including drug treatment, is crucial.

In the past decade, a large number of guidelines for cardiovascular disease prevention have been developed by professional organisations and national societies to guide health professionals. These guidelines have incorporated evidence from landmark clinical trials to produce 'evidence-based' recommendations as well as using other lines of evidence – epidemiological studies, clinical experimentation and expert judgement.

Most guidelines recommend thresholds (when to start treatment) and target levels for certain modifiable risk factors (Box 1.6) and using therapies for achieving these goals for individuals at different levels of risk. Reducing low-density lipoprotein cholesterol (LDL-C) and blood pressure are the most frequently recommended treatment goals.

Specific populations

Guidelines that account for different populations are key as various non-modifiable factors may strongly influence an individual's cardiovascular risk. Factors such as age and sex are well established as influencing an individual's risk. Ethnicity is also important: specific factors confer additional cardiovascular risk, for example, in migrant South Asians the combination of genetics and acquired insulin resistance promotes the metabolic syndrome and increases vascular risk.

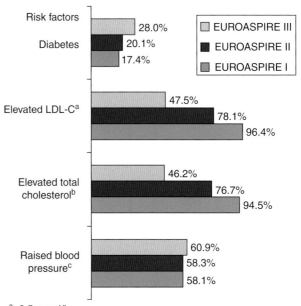

a >2.5 mmol/L
b >4.5 mmol/L
c >140/90 mmHg or > 130/80 mmHg in diabetes patients

Figure 1.5 Results of the EUROASPIRE I, II and III surveys. *Source*: Prevalence of modifiable risk factors in coronary patients interviewed in EUROASPIRE surveys. Ref. 29.

Implementation of guidelines

Successful implementation of risk-reducing strategies remains patchy. The European Action on Secondary Prevention through Intervention to Reduce Events Surveys I and II (EUROASPIRE I and II)[27,28] showed that although 85% of physicians reported using risk assessment tools/guidelines, there was still a high prevalence of modifiable risk factors in coronary patients (Figure 1.5) and inadequate use of prophylactic therapies across

Europe. Results of the EUROASPIRE III survey reported at the European Society of Cardiology 2007 Congress[29] showed that despite impressive increases in the use of cardiovascular medications, smoking levels have remained the same or increased in some groups, body weight has dramatically increased and the prevalence of diabetes has risen since the first survey. Blood pressure management has shown no improvement since the EUROASPIRE surveys started.

EUROACTION is the first pan-European project which aimed to raise the standards of preventive cardiology in Europe by demonstrating that the Joint European Societies' Guidelines on lifestyle, risk factors and therapeutic goals for cardiovascular disease prevention can be realised in everyday clinical practice thus closing the gap between guidelines and practice. The results of EUROACTION showed that a nurse-led multidisciplinary team approach, coupled with the support and involvement of a patient's partner and family, can yield significant improvements in lifestyle and risk factors compared to usual care.[30]

Conclusion

Cardiovascular disease is a major and increasing health issue worldwide. It reduces quality of life and is the commonest cause of premature death in the middle-aged population but is substantially modifiable, with reduction of risk factors proven to reduce cardiovascular events. Guidelines for cardiovascular disease prevention have been developed by professional organisations and national societies to guide health professionals to this goal. However, successful implementation of prevention strategies remains poor.

One reason for the lack of full and effective implementation of official recommendations is reported to be the plethora of guidelines that physicians are confronted within clinical practice. This chapter is the first in a book that aims to provide a practical guide for primary care physicians on the key guidelines on cardiovascular risk management and to illustrate the use of these guidelines.

References

1. Murray CJ, Lopez AD. The global burden of disease: A comprehensive assessment of mortality and disability from diseases, injuries and risk factors in 1990 and projected to 2020. Cambridge, MA,Harvard School of Public Health (Global Burden of Disease and Injury Series, vol. I) 1996.
2. Framingham Heart Study. Available at http://www.framingham-heartstudy.org/about/index.html (Accessed October 2007).
3. Seven Countries Study. Available at http://www.epi.umn.edu/research/7countries/overview.shtm (Accessed October 2007).
4. Tibblin G. High blood pressure in men aged 50. A population study of men born in 1913. *Acta Med Scand*. 1967; 470(Suppl): 1–84
5. Marmot MG, Shipley MJ, Rose G. Inequalities in death – specific explanations of a general pattern? *Lancet*. 1984; 1(8384): 1003–6.
6. Assmann G. Calculating global risk: The key to intervention. *Eur Heart J Suppl*. 2005; 7(Suppl F): F9–F14.
7. MONICA Study. Available at http://www.ktl.fi/monica/index.html (Accessed October 2007).
8. The Cardiovascular Health Study. Available at http://www.chs-nhlbi.org/ (Accessed October 2007).
9. The Rotterdam Study. Available at http://www.epib.nl/ergo.htm (Accessed October 2007).
10. Yusuf S, Hawken S, Ounpuu S, on behalf of the INTERHEART Study Investigators. Effect of potentially modifiable risk factors associated with myocardial infarction in 52 countries (the INTERHEART study): Case-control study. *Lancet*. 2004; 364: 937–52.
11. Rosengren A, Hawken S, Ounpuu S, et al., for the INTERHEART investigators. Association of psychosocial risk factors with risk of acute myocardial infarction in 11 119 cases and 13 648 controls from 52 countries (the INTERHEART study): case-control study. *Lancet*. 2004; 364: 953–62.
12. International Obesity Task Force. EU platform on diet, physical activity and health. March 2005. Available at: http://www.iotf.org/media/euobesity3.pdf (Accessed October 2007).
13. Koek HL, Grobbee DE, Bots ML. Trends in cardiovascular morbidity and mortality in the Netherlands, 1980–2000. *Ned Tijdschr Geneeskd*. 2004; 148(1): 27–32.
14. Stewart S, MacIntyre K, MacLeod MM, et al. Trends in hospitalization for heart failure in Scotland, 1990–1996. An epidemic that has reached its peak? *Eur Heart J*. 2001; 22: 209–17.
15. Mosterd A, Reitsma JB, Grobbee DE. Angiotensin converting enzyme inhibition and hospitalisation rates for heart failure in the Netherlands, 1980–1999: The end of an epidemic? *Heart*. 2002; 87: 75–6.
16. Epstein FH. Cardiovascular disease epidemiology. A journey from the past into the future. *Circulation*. 1996; 93: 1755–64.
17. Heart disease and stroke statistics – 2008 update. A report from the American Heart Association Statistics Committee and Stroke Statistics Subcommittee. *Circulation*. 2008; 117: e25–e146.
18. Petersen S, Peto V, Scarborough P, Rayner M. *Coronary Heart Disease Statistics*. London, BHF, 2005. Available at http://www.heartstats.org/datapage.asp?id=5340.
19. Hennekens CH. Increasing burden of cardiovascular disease: Current knowledge and future directions for research on risk factors. *Circulation*. 1998; 97: 1095–102.
20. ATP III Final Report: II. Rationale for intervention. *Circulation*. 2002; 106: 3163–223.
21. Sleight P, Pouleur H, Zannad F. Benefits, challenges and registerability of the polypill. *Eur Heart J*. 2006; 27(14): 1651–6.
22. Ian Graham, Dan Atar, Knut Borch-Johnsen, Gudrun Boysen, Gunilla Burell, Renata Cifkova, Jean Dallongeville, Guy De Backer, Shah Ebrahim, Bjørn Gjelsvik, Christoph Herrmann-Lingen, Arno Hoes, Steve Humphries, Mike Knapton, Joep Perk, Silia G. Priori, Kalevi Pyorala, Zeljko Reiner, Luis Ruilope, Susana Sans-Menendez, Wilma Scholte op Reimer, Peter Weissberg, David Wood, John Yarnell, Jose Luis Zamorano. European guidelines on cardiovascular disease Prevention in clinical practice: executive summary: Fourth Joint Task Force of the European Society of Cardiology and Other Societies on Cardiovascular Disease Prevention in Clinical Practice (Constituted by representatives of nine societies and by invited experts) *Eur Heart J*. 2007; 28: 2375–2414.
23. Broedl UC, Geiss H-C, Parhofer KG. Comparison of current guidelines for primary prevention of coronary disease. *J Gen Intern Med*. 2003; 18: 190–5.

24. Cullen P, Schulte H, Assmann G. The Münster Heart Study (PROCAM): Total mortality in middle-aged men is increased at low total and LDL cholesterol concentrations in smokers but not in non-smokers. *Circulation*. 1997; 96: 2128–36.

25. Conroy RM, Pyorala K, Fitzgerald AP, Sans S, Menotti A, De Backer G, et al. Estimation of ten-year risk of fatal cardiovascular disease in Europe: The SCORE project. *Eur Heart J*. 2003; 24(11): 987–1003.

26. Graham IM. Guidelines on cardiovascular disease prevention in clinical practice: The European perspective. *Curr Opin Cardiol*. 2005; 20(5): 430–9.

27. EUROASPIRE II Study Group. Lifestyle and risk factor management and use of drug therapies in coronary patients from 15 countries. Principal results from EUROASPIRE II Euro Heart Survey Programme. *Eur Heart J*. 2001; 22: 554–72.

28. EUROASPIRE I and II Groups. Clinical reality of coronary prevention guidelines: A comparison of EUROASPIRE I and II in nine countries. *Lancet*. 2001; 357: 995–1001.

29. Nainggolan L. EUROASPIRE uninspiring: Obesity and smoking wipe out any gains. *Heartwire*, 4 September 2007. Available at http://www.medscape.com/viewarticle/562377 (Accessed October 2007).

30. Clappers N, Verheught FWA. Hotline sessions of the 28th European Congress of Cardiology/World Congress of Cardiology 2006. *Eur Heart J*. 2006; 27(23): 2896–9.

2 Using guidelines as a framework for cardiovascular risk management: comparison of international recommendations

S. Wells[1], E. Washbrook[2] and L. Erhardt[3]

[1]University of Auckland, Auckland, New Zealand
[2]The Future Forum Secretariat, London, UK
[3]Malmö University Hospital, Malmö, Sweden

Introduction

> **Burden of cardiovascular disease**
>
> - Cardiovascular disease accounts for 30% of all deaths and is the leading global cause of morbidity and mortality.
> - During the past two decades, there has been much progress, mostly in the industrialised world, in the management of risk factors for cardiovascular disease.
> - However, the rapidly increasing prevalence of diabetes and obesity in these countries, coupled with the increasing number of people who are adopting sedentary lifestyles and unhealthy diets, threaten to stall or even reverse these gains.

Many national and local groups have developed clinical practice guidelines for cardiovascular risk assessment and management. They aim to consider the relevant evidence and provide practitioners with a framework to identify, risk-assess and manage at-risk individuals according to total cardiovascular risk score, or at a given threshold level of a risk factor. The plethora of available guidelines with sometimes divergent recommendations can itself be a barrier to improving cardiovascular risk management.[1] This series aims to provide practitioners with a clear and concise reference guide to the most cited guidelines developed by expert groups in different regions of the world (Box 2.1).[2-9]

Identification of at-risk patients

Cardiovascular risk assessment and management is applicable to a large proportion of patients seen in primary care. For example, it is estimated that approximately 70% of the New Zealand population over 35 years would meet the national criteria for risk screening.[10] This represents a large proportion of patients seen in daily clinical care. Whilst there is no

randomised control trial evidence to support formal cardiovascular risk screening programmes, there is strong evidence for identifying and treating people at high risk.

Cardiovascular risk factors

Cardiovascular risk factors and recommended treatment options in these guidelines are summarised in Figure 2.1. The major risk factors for cardiovascular disease are considered to be age, gender, smoking, blood pressure, dyslipidaemia (usually related to cholesterol fractions), diabetes and a prior history of ischaemic cardiovascular disease. However some guidelines also include other personal or familial factors (e.g. ethnicity, family history of premature cardiovascular disease), physical or physiological factors (e.g. obesity, impaired glucose tolerance), behavioural factors (e.g. atherogenic diet, physical inactivity) and take into account psychosocial factors (e.g. depression, social isolation, socio-economic deprivation).

Calculation of total cardiovascular disease risk

> **Total cardiovascular disease risk**
>
> - Traditionally we think of cardiovascular disease prevention as 'primary' and 'secondary', or for example, treatment of a patient who is hypertensive or glucose intolerant.
> - This does not fit with the idea of total cardiovascular risk management.
> - Instead, patients should be managed based on their total cardiovascular risk rather than the baseline value of an individual risk factor.
> - Risk is continuous and there is no precise level for blood pressure and cholesterol or glucose below which risk is insignificant.
> - Each individual risk factor contributes to the total cardiovascular risk in a multiplicative way.

Cardiovascular Risk Management, Edited by R Hobbs and B Arroll
© 2009 Blackwell Publishing, ISBN: 9781405155755

Box 2.1 Key regional guidelines for cardiovascular risk management

Australia

Practical Implementation Taskforce for the Prevention of Cardiovascular Disease (2004)
Prevention of cardiovascular disease: An evidence-based clinical aid.
Med J Aust. 2004; 181: F1–F14.
http://www.mja.com.au/public/issues/181_06_200904/ful10382_fm.html

Canada

Working Group on Hypercholesterolaemia and Other Dyslipidaemias (2003)
Recommendations for the management of dyslipidaemia and the prevention of cardiovascular disease: 2003 update.
Genest J, Frohlich J, Fodor G, McPherson R. *CMAJ* 2003; 169: 921–4.
http://www.cmaj.ca/cgi/content/full/169/9/921/DC1.

Europe

Fourth Joint European Task Force (2007)
European guidelines on cardiovascular disease prevention in clinical practice.
Executive Summary: Graham I, Atar AE, Borch-Johsen K, et al. *Eur Heart J.* 2007; 28: 2375–414.
Full text: Graham I, Atar AE, Borch-Johsen K, et al. *Eur J Cardiovasc Prev Rehabil.* 2007; 14(Suppl 2): S1–S113.
http://www.escardio.org/knowledge/guidelines/CVD_Prevention_in_Clinical_Practice.htm

New Zealand

The New Zealand Guidelines Group (2003)
The assessment and management of cardiovascular risk.
http://www.nzgg.org.nz/index.cfm?fuseaction=fuseaction_10&fusesubaction=docs&documentid=22

United Kingdom

Joint British Societies JBS 2 (2005)
Joint British Societies guidelines on prevention of cardiovascular disease in clinical practice. *Heart.* 2005; 91(Suppl V): v1–v52.

United States

National Cholesterol Education Program (2001, 2004)
Third report of the National Cholesterol Education Program (NCEP) expert panel on detection, evaluation, and treatment of high blood cholesterol in adults (Adult Treatment Panel III) (2001).
Expert Panel on detection, evaluation, and treatment of high blood cholesterol in adults. *JAMA.* 2001; 285: 2486–97.
2004 update – Implications of Recent Clinical Trials for the National Cholesterol Education Program Adult Treatment Panel III Guidelines.
Grundy SM, Cleeman JI, Bairey CN, et al. *Circulation.* 2004; 110: 227–39.
http://www.nhlbi.nih.gov/guidelines/cholesterol/index.htm

International
International Atherosclerosis Society (IAS) (2003)
Harmonised guidelines on prevention of atherosclerotic cardiovascular diseases.
http://www.athero.org/

Calculating a patient's risk has been likened to doing your tax return in your head: without a calculator or assessment tool, it will be inaccurate and doctors will fail to identify individuals at high risk. Risk assessment tools (e.g. Systematic Coronary Risk Evaluation (SCORE) or Framingham Heart Study risk equations) combine multiple risk factors to arrive at a score or probability of a coronary or cardiovascular event in a defined time (absolute risk). Unfortunately, guidelines differ with respect to what risk they calculate for example cardiovascular disease death (SCORE) or a combination of coronary heart disease death and non-fatal events (Framingham), which creates confusion. In addition, there is disagreement as to which factors should be included in the algorithms, and the weighting that should be applied to them. However, despite this, these tools are much more accurate at predicting actual future events than not using them at all.

Which risk assessment tool?

- From a practical point of view, it is probably less important which risk assessment calculator or tool is used than not risk scoring at all.
- All risk scores are variations on the same theme; though use differing base data to inform risk calculations.
- All risk scores predict the probability, within a specific time frame, of a significant cardiovascular event for an individual.
- The key message is to use some form of risk assessment as it has been demonstrated that clinical knowledge of the calculated risk leads to better patient management.

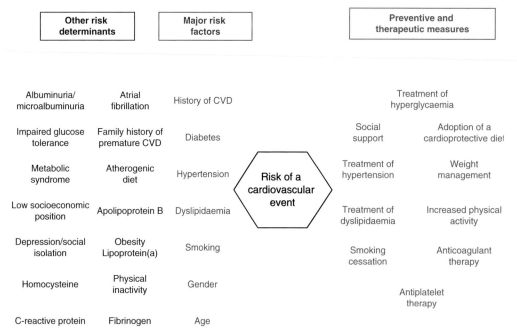

Figure 2.1 Holistic risk management for prevention of cardiovascular disease.

Risk management

There has been a shift away from management based solely on individual risk factors to management based on total cardiovascular risk. Underlying principles are that individuals should have their cardiovascular risk reviewed periodically and managed over their lifetime. Intervention strategies are then tailored according to a patient's short- to medium-term risk: the higher the risk, the greater the intensity of management in order to achieve associated target risk or risk factor levels. For example, early introduction of lifestyle management (cardioprotective dietary patterns, smoking cessation, physical activity programmes) for those adults at low to moderate risk, and concomitant lifestyle and pharmacotherapy for those at high risk.

Actual treatment protocols are still mainly guided to specific targets for individual risk factors rather than to a composite risk score. Drug treatment for those at high cardiovascular risk appears to include a generally well-accepted suite of medications (aspirin, lipid- and blood pressure-lowering drugs).

Although based largely on the same epidemiological evidence, guidelines may differ from each other in their determination of which patient is at 'high risk'. One example is the classification of a patient with diabetes as having equivalent risk (or otherwise) to a patient with a previous cardiovascular event. Similarly there remains uncertainty over the most cost-effective age or risk profile at which to consider commencing primary cardiovascular disease prevention in adults.[11]

Estimation of lifetime risk (e.g. allowing a current risk profile forwarded to the age of 60 or 70 years) has been suggested for younger adults who have a low current absolute risk but who could face a significant shortening of their lifespan unless they achieve changes in their risk factors. However guideline recommendations of drug treatment for younger adults at low current cardiovascular risk who have an unhealthy risk profile, such as smoking, borderline hypertension and mild dyslipidaemia, is to a large extent a societal decision reflecting differing health systems, health policy and fiscal environments. Furthermore, estimated lifetime risk would be high for almost everybody making it almost impossible to target a high-risk group requiring intensive interventions now. The latest 2007 update of the Fourth Joint European Task Force prevention guidelines includes relative risk scores for young people in an attempt to better clarify their risk which, as a result of their young age, is low in absolute terms.

Finally, it needs to be emphasised that managing patients based on any risk algorithm requires a significant portion of clinical judgement.[12] Risk scoring tables never include all factors that confer risk and therefore the physician has to use the calculated risk only as a guide to treatment rather than a reason to treat. Consequently, we should not treat patients based only on the 'number of risks' and all management needs to be individually decided in partnership with the patient.

Whatever the national definition of a high-risk patient (or which patients meet specified criteria for treatment) and despite the general acceptance of guidelines, an alarming proportion of the high-risk population remains unidentified and untreated.[13] Furthermore, many patients who do receive treatment fail to achieve the possible target risk reduction. For example, the results of EUROASPIRE III survey showed that despite impressive increases in the use of all classes of antihypertensive therapies, except calcium-channel blockers, in the 12 years since EUROASPIRE surveys started.[14] The lack of improvement in outcome is likely to be due to increases in some risk factors in survey participants: smoking levels remained the same or increased in some groups, body weight dramatically increased and the prevalence of diabetes rose from 17% in the first survey to 28%.

Benefits of drug treatment[15]

- Using data from trials or meta-analyses of trials it has been estimated that risk of myocardial infarction can be reduced by treatment with
  - Diuretic/beta-blocker: ~20%
  - ACE inhibitor: ~20%
  - Aspirin: ~25%
  - Lipid lowering with statins: ~30%
- Combined relative risk reduction with all four treatments was estimated to be ~70%

Current guidelines from different regions of the world

Australian Practical Implementation Taskforce

These Australian guidelines (Box 2.1) were developed in 2004 by a multidisciplinary group of physicians with the aim of providing an integrated approach to prevention of vascular events, and some key features are summarised in Box 2.2. A one-page chart is provided for use as a desktop reference (Figure 2.2).

Canadian Working Group

In 2000 the Working Group on Hypercholesterolaemia and other Dyslipidaemias issued recommendations for the management of dyslipidaemia. The 2003 guideline update (Boxes 2.1 and 2.3) reflects new clinical trial data and the increasing interest in the metabolic syndrome. The role of risk factors such as apolipoprotein-B and C-reactive protein in risk assessment and use of non-invasive tests (e.g. ankle–brachial index and carotid B-mode ultrasonography) are also discussed.

Fourth Joint European Task Force

In the 1990s, three European societies set up a taskforce to develop guidelines for prevention of coronary heart disease in clinical practice. The taskforce (now comprising nine European societies) issued their most recent guidelines in 2007 (Boxes 2.1 and 2.4). These guidelines recommend using the

---

Box 2.2 Australian guidelines

Practical Implementation Taskforce for the Prevention of Cardiovascular Disease (2004)
Prevention of cardiovascular disease: an evidence-based clinical aid.

- **Target population for risk assessment**: Not clearly defined.

- **Risk calculator**: Use of a risk calculator is recommended; either Framingham Heart Study Prediction Score Sheets, New Zealand Cardiovascular Risk Factor Calculator, or for type 2 diabetes, the UK Prospective Diabetes Study risk calculator.

- **Risk factors identified**:
  - Age
  - Gender
  - Smoking
  - Total choleste rol (TC)
  - HDL-C
  - Blood pressure
  - Proteinuria
  - Depression and social isolation

- **Definition of high risk**:
  - Established coronary, peripheral arterial or cerebrovascular disease
  - Diabetes
  - Renal disease
  - Annual risk of vascular event 2–3% per year or greater

- **Treatment recommendations**:
  - Lifestyle modification for all patients including smoking cessation, physical activity, healthy dietary choices
  - **Total cholesterol threshold for treatment**:
    ○ High-risk patients: TC>3.5 mmol/L or >5.0 mmol/L, depending on disease status
    ○ Low-risk patients: TC>8 mmol/L
  - **Lipid goals**: Not given
  - **Blood Pressure threshold for treatment**:
    ○ High-risk patients: Treat all patients with previous CHD or cerebrovascular disease irrespective of BP, patients with diabetes and BP> 130/85 mmHg, all other high-risk patients with BP>140/90 mmHg.
    ○ Low-risk patients: >150/95 mmHg

- **Blood pressure goals**: Not given

SCORE risk calculator, derived from European studies, to predict the 10-year risk of a fatal cardiovascular event. SCORE accounts for the heterogeneity across Europe by providing separate charts for low- and high-risk regions. It is recommended that each country should develop its own risk charts to allow for the time trends in both mortality and risk factor distribution in individual countries. Information on relative risk as well as absolute risk has been included in the recommendations to facilitate counselling of younger people whose low absolute risk may conceal a substantial and modifiable age-related cardiovascular risk.

The New Zealand Guidelines Group (NZGG)

The New Zealand guidelines were developed in 2003 and have been endorsed by 10 national societies (Boxes 2.1 and 2.5).

Prevention of cardiovasular disease: An evidence-based clinical aid*

	PATIENT RISK CATEGORY					
	High risk					Low risks[§]
TREATABLE RISK FACTORS	Clinically evident coronary heart disease ▪ Previous AMI[†] ▪ Chronic stable angina	Clinically evident cerebrovascular disease Peripheral vascular disease	Diabetes[†‡]	Renal disease	Other risks[§] including ▪ Familial hypercholesterolaemia ▪ Low levels of HDL cholesterol	
Smoking	All smokers should be provided with an active cessation program + medication assistance, if appropriate					
Physical inactivity Obesity	Diet low in saturated fat: increased physical activity (3 × 10 minutes daily): limit excessive alcohol consumption. Target body mass index (BMI) < 25 kg/m², waist < 80 cm for women and < 94 cm for men: waist: hip ratio < 1.[2,3]					
Normal BP (<140/90 mmHg)[3]	ACE inhibitor (ramipril, titrate to 10 mg)[§4]	ACE inhibitor (ramipril, titrate to 10 mg)[§4] Preindopril 4mg+ indapamide 2.5 mg (cerebrovascular disease)[25]	BP < 130/85 [5] Observation, with repeated measurements annually [2,3,5]	BP < 130/85 [5] Observation, with repeated measurements 6 monthly [2,3,5]	Observation, with repeated measurements annually [2,3,5]	Observation, with repeated measurements every 5 years if < 60 years, every 2 years if > 60 years [2,3,5]
High BP (≥140/90 mm HG)[3]	BP > 130/85 [5] ACE inhibitor (ramipril, titrate to 10 mg)[§4] ACE inhibitor[§] [4,6,7,8,9,10,11] Non-ISA b-blocker[†] [5,12,13,14,15] Calcium channel blocker [5,11,12,16,17] Diuretic (thiazide) [4,11,12]	ACE inhibitor (ramipril, titrate to 10 mg)[§4] b-Blocker [5,12,26,27] Diuretic (thiazide) [5,12,26,27] Perindopril 4 mg + indapamide 2.5 mg (cerebrovascular disease)[25]	BP > 130/85 [5] ACE inhibitor[§] [28,29] (ramipril, titrate to 10 mg)[§4] b-Blocker** [5,12] Calcium channel blocker (2nd-line therapy to ACE inhibitor) [5,12,16,17,30,31] Diuretic (thiazide)** [5,12]	BP > 130/85 [§] [4,26,34,35] b-Blocker [5,12] Calcium channel blocker (used with an ACE inhibitor) [30] Diuretic (thiazide) [5,12]	ACE inhibitor [3,5,11,12] b-Blocker [3,5,12] Calcium channel blocker (2nd-line therapy) [5,11,12,16,17] Diuretic (thiazide) [5,11,12]	Drug therapy if: ▪ Systolic BP > 180 or diastolic BP > 100[2] ▪ Systolic BP > 160 or age > 60 years[36] ▪ BP > 140/90 with end-organ damage and/or subclinical disease (microalbuminuria, ST/T wave changes on ECG, left ventricular hypertrophy retinopathy)[2,5,12]
Dyslipidaemia	TC > 3.5 mmol/L Simvastatin 40 mg[21] TC > 4.0 mmol/L Pravastatin 40 mg [3,18,19] or Low HDL-C/high TG Fibrate (gemfibrozil)[22]	TC > 3.5 mmol/L Simvastatin 40 mg[21] TC > 4.0 mmol/L Pravastatin 40 mg [3,18,19] or Low HDL-C/high TG Fibrate (gemfibrozil)[22]	TC > 3.5 mmol/L Simvastatin 40 mg[21] TC > 5.0 mmol/L Statin [3,18,19] Low HDL-C/high TG Fibrate (gemfibrozil)[22] ACE inhibitor (ramipril, titrate to 10 mg)[§4]	TC > 5.0 mmol/L Statin[3] Low HDL-C/high TG Fibrate (gemfibrozil)[3]	TC > 5.0 mmol/L Statin[3] Low HDL-C/high TG Fibrate (gemfibrozil)[3]	TC > 6.0 mmol/L Statin, if lifestyle changes ineffectve[3] TC > 7.5 mmol/L Consider diagnosis of familial hypercholesterolaemia: also secondary causes, other risk factors, and low HDL-C/high TG levels
Proteinuria/ microalbuminuria	Check for diabetes or other causes if evdient: ACE inhibitor (cardiovascular and renal risk reduction) (ramipril, titrate to 10 mg)[§4] ACE inhibitor (renal risk reduction)[23,24]	Check for diabetes or other causes if evdient: ACE inhibitor (cardiovascular and renal risk reduction) (ramipril, titrate to 10 mg)[§4] ACE inhibitor (renal risk reduction)[23,24]	ACE inhibitor (cardiovascular and renal risk reduction) (ramipril, titrate to 10 mg)[§4] ACE inhibitor or irbesartan 300 mg (renal risk reduction) [30,32,33]	Check for diabetes or other causes If > 1g proteinuria: ACE inhibitor [4,23,34,35] Observation, with repeated measurements 6 monthly, if positive	Check for diabetes or other causes if evdient: ACE inhibitor [23,32] Observation, with repeated measurements annually, if positive	Check for diabetes or other causes, as may represent a high-risk group Observation, with repeated measurements annually, if positive

OTHER INTERVENTIONS	
Anti-platelet therapies	Aspirin 75 mg for all patients at high risk of cadiovascular disease.[37,38] Ensure that blood pressure is controlled to minimise risk of haemorrhagic stroke.[39,40] Alternative or additional anti-platelet therapy if aspirin not tolerated, or recurrent coronary heart disease/cerebrovascular disease events occur (dipyridamole, aspirin/dipyridamole, clopidogrel) [20,41,42]
Anticoagulation	Consider in patients with paroxysmal atrial fibrillation: chronic atrial fibrillation: prior thromboembolic event: proteinuria > 3g/day:[43] large anterior myocardial infarction: left ventricular aneurysm: intracardia thrombus: or severe congestive cardiac failure

Reference key

▪ Evidence from meta-analyses or Cochrane Collaboration reviews.

▪ Evidence from meta-analyses or Cochrane Collaboration reviews extrapolated subgroup.

▪ Supported by Australian or international guidelines or peer published opinion.

Specific references are given when there is evidence from meta-analyses or Cochrane Collaboration reviews relating to that particular patient subgroup. When evidence relating to a specific subgroup is not available, general evidence is extrapolated to the subgroup, or references to guidelines or supporting documentation are given.

AMI = acute myocardial infarction
ACE inhibitor = angiotensin-converting enzyme inhibitor
BP = blood pressure
ECG = electrocardiogram
non-ISA = non-intrinsic sympathomimetic activity
TC = total cholesterol
HDL-C = high-density lipoprotein cholesterol
TG = triglycerides

Prevention of cardiovascular disease: an evidence-based clinical aid is intended as a guide for the management of vascular disease, integrating current local and international guidelines and clinical trial data. It should only be used in conjunction with the most recent published guidelines. Therapeutic choices are listed in alphabetical order and not by treatment priority, as this may differ for individual patients. Thresholds are referenced to current guidelines and indicate the level for commencement of therapy. Targets that should be aimed for by applying the recommended intervention are not given.

† Hypertensive and normotensive patients after AMI should receive non-ISA β-blockers. [13–15] There is evidence that, for patients who cannot take β-blockers, non-dihydropyridine calcium channel blockers may be beneficial. [44,45,46]

‡ Fasting blood sugar (≥ 8 hours after consumption of food) ≥ 7.0 mm/L or non-fasting, ≥ 11.1 mmol/L.[1] These blood sugar levels suggest the possibility of diabetes: however single estimations between 5.5 hours and 11.1 mmol/L require confirmation and/or a gluose tolerance test to confirm the diagnosis of diabetes. Routine management of diabetes will include attention to diet ± oral hypoglycaemic agents or insulin. Evidence that intensive glycaemic control will reduce macrovascular events is limited.

§ A patient's risk level is assessed using tools such as the Framingham calculator <http://www.nhlbi.nih/gov.about/framingham/riskabs.htm>. Family history may also modify assessment of a patient's risk. In addition, there is strong evidence of an independencal and causal association between depression, social isolation and the prognosis of coronary heart disease, with the impact of these psychosocial factors being of a similar order to conventional risk factors such as smoking. It is therefore crucial that these factors are considered during individual coronary heart disease risk assessment. In circumstances in which a patient is in more than one risk category, a hieararchical approach (left to right) should be adopted.

¶ See titration schedule in the HOPE study.

**May interfere with diabetic control.

Figure 2.2 Clinical aid chart from the Australian Practical Implementation Taskforce guidelines. *Source*: Reproduced with permission from The Medical Journal of Australia. © Copyright 2004. Ref. 2. (Superscript numbers are citations referenced with Australian Guidelines)

<table>
<tr><td>

Box 2.3 Canadian guidelines

 Working Group on Hypercholesterolaemia and Other Dyslipidaemias (2003)
Recommendations for the management of dyslipidaemia and the prevention of cardiovascular disease: 2003 update

- **Target population for risk assessment:**
  – Men > 40 years, women who are postmenopausal or > 50 years.
  – Individuals with diabetes mellitus, risk factors, or evidence of symptomatic or asymptomatic atherosclerosis.
  – Patients of any age at the discretion of the physician, particularly when lifestyle changes are indicated.

- **Risk calculator:** Framingham Heart Study equation (as per NCEP ATPIII – 10-year CHD risk algorithm).

- **Risk factors identified:**

  – Age
  – Gender
  – Smoking
  – Total cholesterol
  – HDL-C

  – Blood pressure
  – Metabolic syndrome
  – Abdominal obesity
  – Apolipoprotein B, lipoprotein(a), homocysteine or C-reactive protein
  – Genetic factors

- **Definition of high risk:**
  – Established coronary, peripheral arterial or cerebrovascular disease
  – Patients with chronic renal disease
  – Patients with diabetes
  – 10-year risk of CHD event ⩾ 20%

- **Treatment recommendations:**
  – Lifestyle modification – all patients dietary and therapeutic lifestyle changes
  – Concomitant lipid lowering therapy for high-risk patients
  – **Lipid goals:**
    ○ High-risk patients: LDL-C< 2.5 mmol/L and TC/HDL<4 mmol/L
    ○ Moderate-risk patients: LDL-C < 3.5 mmol/L and TC/HDL<5 mmol/L
    ○ Low-risk patients: LDL-C < 4.5 mmol/L and TC/HDL<6 mmol/L
  – **Blood pressure:**
    ○ No targets or advice provided

</td><td>

Box 2.4 European guidelines

 Fourth Joint European Task Force (2007)
European guidelines on cardiovascular disease prevention in clinical practice

- **Target population for risk assessment:**
  – Patients with established atherosclerotic cardiovascular disease.
  – Asymptomatic individuals at high risk of atherosclerotic CVD (including patients with diabetes or multiple risk factors).
  – Close relatives of patients with early onset CVD disease or of asymptomatic people at particularly high risk.
  – Other individuals encountered in routine clinical practice.

- **Risk calculator:** SCORE (10-year risk of fatal CVD events)

- **Risk factors identified:**

  – Age
  – Gender
  – Smoking
  – Total cholesterol, LDL-C, triglycerides
  – HDL-C
  – Blood pressure
  – Diabetes/impaired glucose tolerance
  – Nutrition

  – Inflammatory markers/ haemostatic factors
  – Family history of premature CVD/genetics
  – Preclinical atherosclerosis (e.g. detected by CT scan, ultrasonography)
  – Obesity/overweight
  – Physical activity level
  – Psychosocial factors
  – Renal impairment

- **Definition of high risk:**
  – Established atherosclerotic cardiovascular disease
  – Type 2 diabetes and Type 1 diabetes with microalbuminuria
  – 10-year risk of fatal CVD event ⩾ 5%

- **Treatment recommendations:**
  – Lifestyle modifications for all patients including smoking cessation, physical activity, healthy dietary choices.
  – Consider concomitant drug therapy (aspirin, lipid lowering, BP lowering) for high-risk patients.
  – **LDL-C goals:**
    ○ Patients with established CVD or diabetes: LDL-C < 2.5 mmol/L (~100 mg/dL).
    ○ Other patients: LDL-C < 3.0 mmol/L (115 mg/dL)
  – **Blood pressure goals:**
    ○ High-risk patients: <140/90 mmHg
    ○ Diabetic patients: <130/80 mmHg

</td></tr>
</table>

Framingham-based risk tables are used, yielding 5-year risk of a fatal or non-fatal cardiovascular event. As Framingham risk prediction may underestimate the risk in certain patient groups, these guidelines recommend an upward risk adjustment (an additional 5% 5-year cardiovascular risk) for Maori, Pacific people and those from the Indian subcontinent, people with family history of premature ischaemic cardiovascular disease, metabolic syndrome, patients with diabetes and microalbuminuria and Type 2 diabetes for more than 10 years duration or with

an HbA1c consistently over 8%. Treatment decisions based on 5-year risk are summarised in a flow chart (Figure 2.3).

Joint British Societies' Guidelines

In 1998 the Joint British Societies published recommendations on prevention of coronary heart disease in clinical practice. A key change in the 2005 update (Boxes 2.1 and 2.6) is the broadening of scope to prevention of atherosclerotic cardiovascular disease with estimation of fatal and non-fatal cardiovascular

---

Box 2.5 New Zealand guidelines

The New Zealand Guidelines Group (2003)
The assessment and management of cardiovascular risk

- **Target population**:
  - All men > 45 years, women > 55 years and 10 years earlier for Maori, Pacific or Indian subcontinent.
  - Patients who have other known CVD risk factors or at high risk of developing diabetes.

- **Risk calculator**: Framingham 5-year fatal and non-fatal CVD risk

- **Risk factors identified**:

– Age	– Type 2 diabetes of	– Physical inactivity
– Gender	long duration or	– Family history of premature CVD
– Smoking	HbA1c consistently	– Low socioeconomic position
– Total cholesterol,	over 8%	– Depression and social isolation
triglycerides	– Atrial fibrillation	– Apolipoprotein B, C-reactive
– HDL-C	– Abdominal obesity	protein, microalbuminuria,
– Blood pressure	– Impaired glucose regulation/	lipoprotein(a), homocysteine or
– Diabetes	metabolic syndrome	fibrinogen
– Diabetes and	– Poor nutritional pattern	

- **Definition of high risk**:
  - Previous cardiovascular event, certain genetic lipid disorders
  - Diabetes and renal disease
  - 5-year risk of CVD event ⩾ 15%
  - Patients with total cholesterol ⩾8, TC:HDL ratio ⩾8 or BP⩾170/100

- **Treatment recommendations**:
  - Lifestyle modification for all patients including smoking cessation, physical activity, healthy dietary choices
  - Concomitant drug therapy (aspirin, lipid lowering, BP lowering) for high-risk patients
  - **LDL-C goals**:
    - Patients following venous coronary artery bypass grafting <2 mmol/L
    - All others: <2.5 mmol/L
  - **Blood pressure goals**:
    - Patients with diabetes or CVD: < 130/80 mmHg
    - All others: <140/85 mmHg

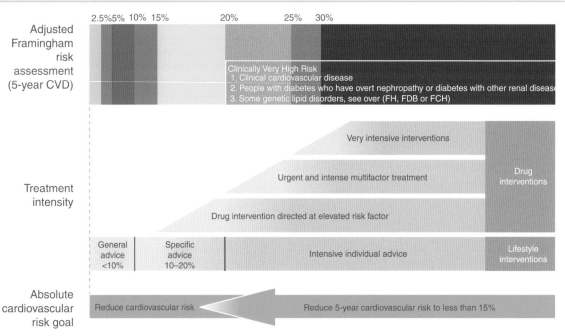

Figure 2.3 Treatment decisions based on 5-year cardiovascular risk from the NZGG guidelines. The higher the person's absolute risk of a cardiovascular event, the more aggressively modifiable risk factors should be managed. *Source*: Reproduced with permission from New Zealand Guidelines Group. The Assessment and Management of Cardiovascular Risk. An Evidence-Based Best Practice Guideline. Wellington, NZ, 2003. www.nzgg.org.nz (Ref. 5; http://www.nzgg.org.nz/guidelines/0035/CVD_Risk_Full.pdf).

Box 2.6 United Kingdom guidelines

 Joint British Societies' Guidelines (2005)
JBS 2 Prevention of cardiovascular disease in clinical practice

- **Target population:**
  - All adults over 40 years and younger adults with a family history of premature atherosclerotic disease

- **Risk calculator:** Framingham 10-year fatal and non-fatal CVD risk

- **Risk factors identified:**
  - Age
  - Gender
  - Smoking
  - Total cholesterol, triglycerides
  - HDL-C
  - Blood pressure
  - Diabetes
  - Family history of premature CVD
  - Abdominal obesity
  - Impaired glucose regulation
  - Women with premature menopause
  - Poor nutritional pattern
  - Physical inactivity
  - Low socioeconomic position
  - Depression and social isolation
  - Apolipoprotein B, C-reactive protein, lipoprotein(a), homocysteine or fibrinogen

- **Definition of high risk:**
  - Any established atherosclerotic CVD
  - Diabetes mellitus (Type 1 or 2)
  - 10-year risk of CVD event ⩾ 20%
  - Familial dyslipidaemia
  - Patients with TC:HDL ratio ⩾6 or BP⩾160/100 mmHg

- **Treatment recommendations:**
  - Lifestyle modification for all patients including smoking cessation, physical activity, healthy dietary choices
  - Concomitant drug therapy (aspirin, lipid lowering, BP lowering) for high-risk patients
- **Primary lipid goals:**
  - Total cholesterol <4 mmol/L and LDL-C< 2.0 mmol/L OR a 25% reduction in total cholesterol and 30% reduction in LDL-C
  - All others: <2.5 mmol/L

- **Blood pressure goals:**
  - Patients with CVD, diabetes or chronic renal failure: <130/80 mmHg
  - All others at high risk: <140/85 mmHg

event risk. Non-fasting glucose is included as part of the initial risk assessment to detect impaired glucose tolerance or new diabetes. Optimal levels of risk factors are given, as well as audit standards, which are considered to be the minimum standard of care for high-risk people. Furthermore these guidelines discuss the need for screening first degree relatives of people with premature cardiovascular disease, organisation of preventive care in hospital and in general practice, integrated patient care between the settings and audit of the care of high-risk patients.

USA Third National Cholesterol Education Program (NCEP)

The Adult Treatment Panel III (ATP III) of NCEP issued guidelines on cholesterol management in 2001 (Boxes 2.1 and 2.7). Individuals are assigned to three risk categories through a combination of counting the number of major risk factors present and the Framingham algorithm to estimate the 10-year risk of a coronary heart disease event. In contrast to the European guidelines, high-density lipoprotein cholesterol (HDL-C) is included in the risk algorithm. The guidelines focus on lifestyle changes and treating dyslipidaemia, in particular LDL-C. The update published in 2004 reviewed the results of five major clinical trials of statin therapy and recommended more aggressive lipid-lowering therapy particularly for those at very high risk.

International Atherosclerosis Society (IAS)

The IAS has integrated several guidelines from international and national organisations to provide a rational strategy that can be adapted for worldwide use (Boxes 2.1 and 2.8). These 'harmonised' guidelines aim to emphasise the major areas of agreement among guidelines and to consider reasons for discrepancies. The IAS guidelines compare the Prospective Cardiovascular Münster study (PROCAM) and Framingham Heart Study algorithms for risk assessment, and consider various approaches to risk assessment in diabetes patients. Tables that clearly summarise the goals and principles of management of major and emerging risk factors are included.

Additional guidelines

This summary is only a selection of the most recent international cardiovascular risk management guidelines. Many others have been published.[16-18] A number of guidelines have been developed solely for management of patients with diabetes (Box 2.9).[19-24] As cardiovascular disease is the major cause of mortality in patients with diabetes it may be beneficial to use these guidelines in conjunction with cardiovascular disease guidelines discussed above.

Implementing guidelines

Implementing cardiovascular risk assessment and management guidelines to realise the potential for reducing the burden of disease requires an organised, coordinated approach within and between hospital and general practice, including team building and systematisation (e.g. alerts at the time of routine consultation, reminders, decision support tools, systematic coding, reporting and auditing of care). Just as important is the development of clinical skills in risk communication, motivational interviewing, care planning and assisting patient self-management. This is discussed in more detail later in the series.

Box 2.7 USA guidelines

National Cholesterol Education Program (2001, 2004)

Third report of the NCEP expert panel on detection, evaluation and treatment of high blood cholesterol in adults (Adult Treatment Panel III) (2001)

2004 update – Implications of Recent Clinical Trials for the National Cholesterol Education Program Adult Treatment Panel III Guidelines

- **Target population**: All adults 20 years or older recommended to have fasting lipid profile

- **Risk calculator^**: Two-step procedure – the number of major risk factors (exclusive of LDL-C) as below are counted. Then those patients with two or more risk factors have 10-year CHD risk calculated with a Framingham score.

- **Risk factors identified**:

Lipid profile (LDL-C, total cholesterol, HDL-C)

Plus following major risk factors counted
- Smoking
- Hypertension (BP≥ 140/90 mmHg or on BP treatment
- Family history of premature coronary heart disease (CHD)

Other risk factors
- Age, gender
- Obesity, Physical inactivity
- Atherogenic diet
- Lipoprotein(a), homocysteine, inflammatory markers and prothrombotic markers
- Impaired fasting glucose/ metabolic syndrome
- Sub-clinical atherosclerotic disease

- **Definition of high risk**:
  - Established CHD, other clinical forms of atherosclerotic disease
  - Diabetes
  - 10-year risk of CHD event > 20%

- **Treatment recommendations**:
  - Lifestyle modification for all patients including smoking cessation, physical activity, healthy dietary choices
  - Concomitant lipid lowering drug therapy for high-risk patients
  - LDL-C goals:
    ○ High-risk patients: <100 mg/dL (2.6 mmol/L)
    ○ Moderate-risk patients (2+ risk factors): <130 mg/dL (3.4 mmol/L)
    ○ Low-risk patients (0–1 risk factors): <160 mg/dL (4.1 mmol/L)
  - Blood pressure:
    ○ No targets or advice provided

Box 2.8 International guidelines

International Atherosclerosis Society (IAS) (2003)

Harmonised guidelines on prevention of atherosclerotic cardiovascular diseases

- **Target population**: Not clearly defined.

- **Risk calculator**: Risk algorithms based on either Framingham or PROCAM studies. Both tools recognised as valid and provide similar but not identical estimates.

- **Risk factors identified**:
  - Atherogenic diet
  - Overweight and obesity
  - Physical inactivity
  - Age
  - Gender
  - Smoking
  - Blood pressure
  - Diabetes
  - LDL-C
  - HDL-C
  - triglycerides
  - Impaired glucose regulation
  - Family history of premature cardiovascular disease
  - Apolipoprotein B, small LDL particles, lipoprotein (a), C-reactive protein, fibrinogen, homocysteine

- **Definition of high risk**:
  - Established CHD plus other clinical forms of non-coronary atherosclerotic disease
  - 10-year risk of CHD event > 20%
  - Diabetes considered a CHD risk equivalent in higher risk populations such as in the United States, where people with diabetes have high average CHD risk (otherwise appropriate to count diabetes as a risk factor and use risk assessment tool.

- **Treatment recommendations**:
  - Lifestyle modification for all patients including smoking cessation, physical activity, healthy dietary choices, management of overweight and obesity
  - LDL-C goals
    ○ High-risk patients: <2.6 mmol/L
    ○ Moderate-risk patients (2+ risk factors): <3.4 mmol/L
    ○ Low-risk patients (0–1 risk factor): <4.1 mmol/L
  - Blood pressure goals:
    ○ High-risk patients: <130/85 mmHg
    ○ Low-risk patients: <140/90 mmHg

- **Guidelines integrated into the IAS guidelines**: Third Report of NCEP ATP, Joint European Cardiovascular Societies, American Heart Association, American College of Cardiology, United States NHLBI for Cholesterol, Blood Pressure and Obesity, International Task Force for Prevention of Coronary Heart Disease, World Health Organization and various national and international societies for hypertension and diabetes

Conclusion

The guidelines presented demonstrate consistency of recommendations in respect of managing individuals identified as being at risk of a cardiovascular event. Recommendations regarding thresholds and interventions for lower risk individuals are less uniform, with variations reflecting national priorities and the fact that cardiovascular risk can be lowered in 'all' patients but the benefits decrease as the risk declines. Most guidelines recommend formal risk assessment using tables or calculators.

Box 2.9 Guidelines for management of patients with diabetes

American Diabetes Association (2007)
2007 Clinical Practice Recommendations. Standards of Medical Care in Diabetes. *Diabetes Care*. 2007;
30(Suppl 1): S3–103.
http://www.diabetes.org/for-health-professionals-and-scientists/cpr.jsp
Compilation of all current American Diabetes Association position statements on the management of patients
with diabetes.

American College of Physicians (2004)
Lipid control in the management of Type 2 diabetes mellitus: a practical guideline from the American College of Physicians.
Snow V, Aronson MD, Hornbake ER, et al. *Ann Intern Med*. 2004; 140: 644–9.
www.annals.org
Guidelines on the management of dyslipidaemia particularly hypercholesterolaemia for patients with Type 2 diabetes.

Diabetes Australia Guidelines Development Consortium (2004)
National evidence based guidelines for the management of Type 2 diabetes mellitus: Prevention and detection of
macrovascular disease.
http://www.diabetes.net.au/PDF/update_04_2004/macrovascular.pdf
Aimed principally at general practitioners to promote the effective and efficient identification of risk factors for CVD
as well as the presence of existing macrovascular disease.

Canadian Diabetes Association Clinical Practice Guidelines Expert Committee (2003)
Clinical Practice Guidelines for the Prevention and Management of Diabetes in Canada. *Can J Diabetes*. 2003;
27(Suppl 2): S1–S152.
http://www.diabetes.ca/cpg2003/default.aspx
Guidelines on the management of diabetes, including cardiovascular risk factors.

International Diabetes Federation Clinical Guidelines Task Force (2005)
Global Guidelines for Type 2 Diabetes.
Brussels: International Diabetes Federation, 2005
http://www.idf.org/home/index.cfm?node=1457
Global guidelines developed using the evidence analyses of prior national and local guidelines. Contains advice on
management of cardiovascular risk factors and CHD.

New Zealand Guidelines Group (2003)
Management of Type 2 Diabetes.
http://www.nzgg.org.nz; ISBN 0-476-00092-0
Includes a dedicated section on management of cardiovascular risk and risk factors.

References

1. Ballantyne C, Arroll B, Shepherd J. Lipids and CVD management: Towards a global consensus. *Eur Heart J*. 2005; 26(21): 2224–31.
2. Prevention of cardiovascular disease: An evidence-based clinical aid. *Med J Aust*. 2004; 181: F1–1.
3. Genest J, Frohlich J, Fodor G, McPherson R. Recommendations for the management of dyslipidemia and the prevention of cardiovascular disease: 2003 update. *CMAJ*. 2003; 169: 921–4.
4. Graham I, Atar AE, Borch-Johsen K et al. European guidelines on cardiovascular disease prevention in clinical practice. *Eur J Cardiovasc Prev Rehabil*. 2007; 14(Suppl 2): S1–113.
5. The assessment and management of cardiovascular risk. Available at http://www.nzgg.org.nz/index.cfm?fuseaction=fuseaction_10&fusesubaction=docs&documentid=22 (Accessed October 2007).
6. Joint British Societies guidelines on prevention of cardiovascular disease in clinical practice. *Heart*. 2005; 91(Suppl V): v1–52.
7. Third report of the National Cholesterol Education Program (NCEP) expert panel on detection, evaluation, and treatment of high blood cholesterol in adults (Adult Treatment Panel III) (2001). Expert panel on detection, evaluation, and treatment of high blood cholesterol in adults. *JAMA*. 2001; 285: 2486–97.
8. Grundy SM, Cleeman JI, Bairey CN et al. 2004 update – Implications of Recent Clinical Trials for the National Cholesterol Education Program Adult Treatment Panel III Guidelines. *Circulation*. 2004; 110: 227–39.
9. International Atherosclerosis Society (IAS) (2003). Harmonized guidelines on prevention of atherosclerotic cardiovascular diseases. Available at http://www.athero.org/ (Accessed October 2007).
10. Wells S, Broad J, Jackson R. Estimated prevalence of cardiovascular disease and distribution of cardiovascular risk in New Zealanders: Data for healthcare planners, funders, and providers. *NZ Med J*. 2006; 119: 1232. Available at: http://www.nzma.org.nz/journal/119-1232/1935/ (Accessed October 2007).
11. Ulrich S, Hingorani AD, Martin J, Vallance P. What is the optimal age for starting lipid lowering treatment? A mathematical model. *BMJ*. 2000; 320(7242): 1134–40.
12. Backlund L, Bring L, Strender LE. How accurately do general practitioners and students estimate coronary risk in hypercholesterolaemic patients? *Prim Health Care Res Dev*. 2004; 5: 153–61.
13. Mosca L, Linfante AH, Benjamin EJ, Berra K, Hayes SN, Walsh BW et al. National study of physician awareness and adherence to cardiovascular disease prevention guidelines. *Circulation*. 2005; 111: 499–510.

14. Nainggolan L. EUROASPIRE uninspiring: obesity and smoking wipe out any gains. Heartwire, 4 September 2007. Available at http://www.medscape.com/viewaticle/562377 (Accessed October 2007).

15. Emberson J, Whincup P, Morris R, Walker M, Ebrahim S. Evaluating the impact of population and high-risk strategies for the primary prevention of cardiovascular disease. *Eur Heart J.* 2004; 25: 484–91.

16. Mosca L, Appel LJ, Benjamin EJ, Berra K, Chandra-Strobos N, Fabunmi RP et al. Evidence-based guidelines for cardiovascular disease prevention in women. American Heart Association scientific statement. *Arterioscler Thromb Vasc Biol.* 2004; 24: e29–50.

17. Smaha LA. American Heart Association. The American Heart Association Get with The Guidelines program. *Am Heart J.* 2004; 148(Suppl 5): S46–8.

18. Smith Jr, SC, Jackson R, Pearson TA, Fuster V, Yusuf S, Faergeman O et al. Principles for national and regional guidelines on cardiovascular disease prevention: A scientific statement from the World Heart and Stroke Forum. *Circulation.* 2004; 109: 3112–21.

19. 2007 Clinical Practice Recommendations. Standards of Medical Care in Diabetes. *Diabetes Care* 2007; 30(Suppl 1): S3–103.

20. Snow V, Aronson MD, Hornbake ER, et al. Lipid control in the management of type 2 diabetes mellitus: A practical guideline from the American College of Physicians. *Ann Intern Med.* 2004; 140: 644–9.

21. National evidence based guidelines for the management of type 2 diabetes mellitus: Prevention and detection of macrovascular disease. Available at http://www.diabetes.net.au/PDF/update_04_2004/macrovascular.pdf (Accessed October 2007).

22. Clinical Practice Guidelines for the prevention and management of diabetes in Canada. *Can J Diabetes.* 2003; 27(Suppl 2): S1–152.

23. Global Guidelines for Type 2 Diabetes. Brussels: International Diabetes Federation, 2005. Available at http://www.idf.org/home/index.cfm?node=1457 (Accessed October 2007).

24. Management of Type 2 Diabetes. Available at http://www.nzgg.org.nz (Accessed October 2007).

3 Identifying high-risk patients

A.W. Hoes[1], E. Washbrook[2] and R. Jackson[3]

[1]University Medical Center Utrecht, Utrecht, The Netherlands
[2]Future Forum Secretariat, London, UK
[3]University of Auckland, Auckland, New Zealand

Introduction

Numerous factors have been identified to be associated with increased risk of incident or recurrent cardiovascular disease (CVD). Such factors are typically referred to as cardiovascular risk factors, or risk indicators as the associations are not necessarily causal. The more commonly cited risk factors are summarised in Table 3.1. Usually only the major risk factors are taken into account when estimating a patient's cardiovascular risk, while the additional predictive value of novel risk indicators in clinical practice remains to be established. Most cardiovascular risk factors are continuous variables (e.g. blood pressure) and risk increases across their usual distributions in western countries. Arbitrary cut-off points have traditionally been used to define these continuous risk factors (e.g. hypertension), but more accurate cardiovascular risk assessment methods are now available that can incorporate specific values.

A patient's absolute cardiovascular risk is determined by the synergistic effect of all risk factors present and so it is necessary to consider all major risk factors when estimating risk.[1,2] Multifactorial risk assessment is difficult to do accurately in one's head and numerous tools are now available to aid clinicians. Moreover, the benefits of interventions are directly proportional to this multifactorial, absolute cardiovascular risk and small abnormalities in multiple risk factors typically result in higher risks than a large abnormality in a single risk factor.[3] This observation has major implications for cardiovascular risk assessment and management practices, and traditional approaches focusing on the assessment and management of hypertension and dyslipidaemia are no longer considered clinically effective or efficient.

Levels of risk

Individuals with established CVD are generally at high risk of a recurrent event whatever their cardiovascular risk factor

Table 3.1 Cardiovascular risk factors*

Major risk factors		Emerging risk factors[a]
Non-modifiable	Modifiable	
Established CVD[b]	Cigarette smoking	Homocysteine
Age	High-saturated fat diet	C-reactive protein
Gender	Body mass index[c]/waist circumference	Albuminuria
Family history of premature coronary heart disease	Physical activity Systolic and diastolic blood pressure LDL-cholesterol HDL-cholesterol Triglycerides Diabetes/blood glucose Socioeconomic status Left ventricular mass	Coagulation factors (e.g. fibrinogen) Other lipid factors (e.g. apolipoproteins) Ankle–brachial index Carotid artery intima media thickness (ultrasonography) Calcifications in the aorta or coronaries (CT scanning or other imaging techniques)

*Does not imply direct causality.
[a]Value in addition to the major risk factors clinical practice for assessing absolute cardiovascular risk remains to be established.
[b]Includes angina, myocardial infarction, angioplasty, coronary artery bypass grafting, transient ischaemic attack, ischaemic stroke or peripheral arterial disease.
[c]Body mass index = weight (kg) per length (m^2).

profile and do not require a multifactorial risk assessment to determine whether they are at high risk. Patients with diabetes are also considered to be at increased cardiovascular risk, but there is considerable controversy regarding their risk level, which apart from their multifactorial risk profile also depends on diabetes-related factors, such as the duration of the condition and renal function. Other patients are considered to be at increased risk for CVD, when the combined effects of their risk factors are such that their multifactorial risk for CVD exceeds stated thresholds. Such thresholds differ across guidelines, but are usually determined by weighing the clinical

Cardiovascular Risk Management, Edited by R Hobbs and B Arroll
© 2009 Blackwell Publishing, ISBN: 9781405155755

benefit, costs and logistic consequences of interventions. In patients without established CVD, risk should be determined using multifactor risk calculators. Typically, only the major risk factors are included in the calculators (i.e. the strongest and easiest to assess) to ensure the applicability of risk calculations in clinical practice.

Many national and local groups have developed guidelines that provide a framework to identify and evaluate patients at increased risk of CVD. This article provides practical guidance on how to effectively identify patients at risk of CVD and assess their level of risk, based on recommendations from key up-to-date cardiovascular guidelines available in English. These recommendations can be simplified to three steps (Figure 3.1).

Step 1: Select people for cardiovascular risk assessment

The purpose of cardiovascular risk assessment is to detect those individuals at increased cardiovascular risk, with the aim of using the estimated risk to guide the intensity of preventative interventions. As discussed above, patients with established CVD do not require a formal absolute risk assessment as their symptomatic disease alone places them at high risk, warranting targeted interventions. Nevertheless, knowledge of their risk levels could guide and improve compliance with prevention strategies such as smoking cessation and physical activity training.

Certain population groups are more likely to be at increased risk than others, such as older people, certain ethnic groups or people with a family history of CVD, and many guideline recommendations prioritise these groups for assessment (Table 3.2). For example, Canadian guidelines recommend screening all men over 40 years and all women above 50 years.[4] The New Zealand guidelines recommend screening Maori, Pacific and people from the Indian subcontinent 10 years earlier than other population groups.[5] Several guidelines recommend that close relatives of patients with premature coronary heart disease (CHD) and people in families with familial hypercholesterolaemia or other inherited dyslipidaemias should also be examined for cardiovascular risk indicators. It should be emphasised that the evidence underlying most of these recommendations is poor and their cost effectiveness has often not been evaluated. No doubt the differences between guidelines are partly attributable to this knowledge gap. Moreover, most guidelines do not state how such

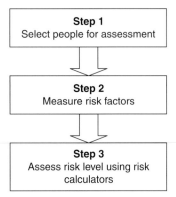

Figure 3.1 Steps in assessment of cardiovascular risk.

Table 3.2 Recommended criteria for CV risk assessment in individuals without CVD

Subgroup	Guideline			
	Canada	Europe	NZ	USA
People without CVD or known risk factors	All >40/>50 years (men/women)	–	All >45/>55 years (men/women)	All >20 years (men/women)
People with cardiovascular risk factors	All with >1 risk factors, diabetes or evidence of atherosclerosis	All with diabetes, multiple risk factors or family history of premature CVD	All >35/>45 years (men/women) with known risk factors or a high risk of diabetes	All >20 years (men/women)
Ethnic groups Maori, Pacific people and people from the Indian subcontinent	–	–	All >35/>45 years (men/women)	–

The International and Australian guidelines do not provide any clearly defined guidance on selecting people for risk assessment.

screening activities should be organised: in primary care hospitals or by government or other organisations.

Step 2: Measure risk factors

Once a patient has been identified for assessment, a comprehensive cardiovascular risk assessment should be carried out, which involves the measurement and recording of all major risk indicators (Box 3.1). As the magnitude of the cardiovascular risk is determined by the synergistic effect of the combined risk factors, it is important to measure all relevant factors.

As discussed above, people with diabetes are usually at higher cardiovascular risk than non-diabetic people with similar risk factor profiles. Prospective studies show that cardiovascular risk is 2–5 times higher than in the population at large, but the magnitude of this increased risk depends on diabetes-related factors, notably the time since diagnosis.[6,7] The assessment of people with diabetes differs between the guidelines. For example, diabetes is not listed in the calculations of the American NCEP and Canadian guidelines as people with diabetes are categorised as 'CHD equivalents'.[4,8,9] Most other guidelines consider diabetes as a risk factor and include it in the risk assessment. The New Zealand guidelines, for example, make a 5% 5-year cardiovascular risk adjustment to patients with diabetes diagnosed more than 10 years previously; this is in addition to the weighting given to diabetes in the Framingham-based risk score.[5]

Some population groups appear to be particularly susceptible to certain risk factors and exhibit higher cardiovascular morbidity and mortality than other groups, despite similar risk profiles. As mentioned earlier, the Maori, Pacific people and people from the Indian subcontinent are identified at increased risk in the New Zealand guidelines and receive an additional 5% 5-year cardiovascular risk weighting.[5] In addition, the American NCEP guidelines identify South Asians as being at increased risk for CVD, and greater attention is recommended for detection of increased cardiovascular risk in this population.[8,9]

The European guidelines also identify national and regional differences, with Europe divided into low- and high-risk countries (Figure 3.2).[10] This has resulted in the European guidelines providing two risk calculators depending on whether the person is from a low- or high-risk region.

Most guidelines also recognise the so-called 'metabolic syndrome', in which clustering of certain cardiovascular risk indicators is associated with increased risk of a cardiovascular event.[11] Three or more of the five risk factors (all continuous variables that have been arbitrarily dichotomised) are required for a diagnosis of metabolic syndrome (Table 3.3). A more appropriate approach would be to develop a metabolic score incorporating the actual levels of these continuous variables.

In addition, certain emerging risk factors and measures of subclinical atherosclerosis (Table 3.1) may be used as adjuncts to the major risk factors in assessing risk, although data on their added value in determining the absolute risk of CVD in daily practice is limited. Assessment of these risk indicators should be limited to special circumstances in which the decision to intervene is uncertain based on standard risk factors.

Step 3: Assess risk level using risk calculators

As discussed, risk assessment in individual patients can be complex because the effects of multiple risk factors interact.

Box 3.1 Risk indicators typically measured and recorded when assessing cardiovascular risk

- Age
- Gender
- Ethnicity*
- Smoking history
- Lipid profile (*Note*: Fasting is unnecessary for total cholesterol or HDL-cholesterol)
- Fasting plasma glucose/diabetes
- Blood pressure
- Family history of premature CVD
- Body mass index/waist circumference
- Left ventricular hypertrophy.

*Not all guidelines take ethnicity into account when assessing risk.

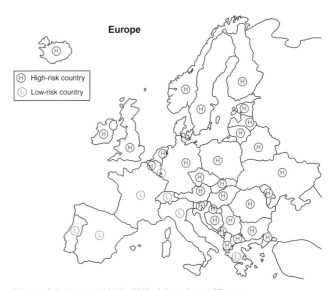

Figure 3.2 Low- and high-CVD risk regions of Europe.

Table 3.3 Clinical identification of the metabolic syndrome, according to the National Cholesterol Education Program (NCEP)

Risk factor	Defining level
Abdominal obesity waist circumference	
Men	>102 cm*
Women	>88 cm*
Triglycerides	>1.7 mmol/L
HDL-cholesterol	
Men	<1.0 mmol/L
Women	<1.3 mmol/L
Blood pressure	>130/85 mmHg
Fasting glucose	>6.1 mmol/L**

*New Zealand guidelines recommend levels of 100 and 90 cm for men and women, respectively.[5]

**Canadian guidelines recommend levels of 6.2–7.0 mmol/L.[4]

Box 3.2 Risk calculators incorporated into cardiovascular guidelines

Framingham

- **Australia:** National Heart Foundation of Australia; The Cardiac Society of Australia and New Zealand. Lipid Management Guideline

- **Canada:** Working Group on Hypercholesterolaemia and other Dyslipidaemias

- **New Zealand:** The New Zealand Guidelines Group, the National Heart Foundation of New Zealand and the Stroke Foundation of New Zealand

- **United States:** Third Report of The National Cholesterol Education Program

- **International:** International Atherosclerosis Society (IAS)

SCORE

- **Europe:** Fourth Joint European Task Force

PROCAM

- **International:** International Atherosclerosis Society (IAS)

To aid this process, a number of risk calculators have been developed (Box 3.2), and are recommended in guidelines.

Although there is some variation between the different calculators,[12,13] the majority are based on logistic regression (or similar) equations. Computer-based tools are the most accurate approach, but risk charts (e.g. Figures 3.3 and 3.4) are reasonable alternatives. The calculators estimate an individual's risk of experiencing a cardiovascular event over a given period of time, usually 10 or 5 years. This time period, as well as the specific outcome (either fatal or the combination of fatal and non-fatal CHD or CVD) varies between calculators.

In most guidelines, risk determined by risk calculators is usually categorised as high-, intermediate- and low-risk. The definitions of these categories given by different guidelines are summarised in Table 3.4. Higher risk demands more intensive intervention and stricter treatment goals. Treatment decisions are adjusted according to an individual's risk category (see the following articles in this series on management recommendations).

Risk calculators

The most widely used risk calculators are based on the Framingham Heart Study,[14] the SCORE project,[15] PROCAM[16] and UKPDS.[17–20] The studies that each risk calculator system is based on are summarised in Table 3.5.

Data from the Framingham Heart Study, a long-term follow up of approximately 5,000 men and women from Framingham, Massachusetts, United States, with both fatal and non-fatal cardiovascular endpoints have been used as the basis of many risk prediction systems, but tend to overestimate risk in some European and non-European populations.[14] More recently, charts predicting fatal CVD were created using data from the SCORE project designed to improve prediction in European countries.[15] SCORE involved individuals with no evidence of pre-existing CVD from 12 European cohort studies, across multiple countries. Importantly, statistical techniques are available for adjusting risk scores, taking into account the incidence of CVD and mean level of the main risk factors in individual countries. The SCORE calculator provides specific guidelines on how to achieve this.

Available formats for risk calculators

The risk calculators are available as risk charts, computer-assisted algorithms (including neural network analysis) and spreadsheets to assist practitioners in office-based assessment of patients (Box 3.3).

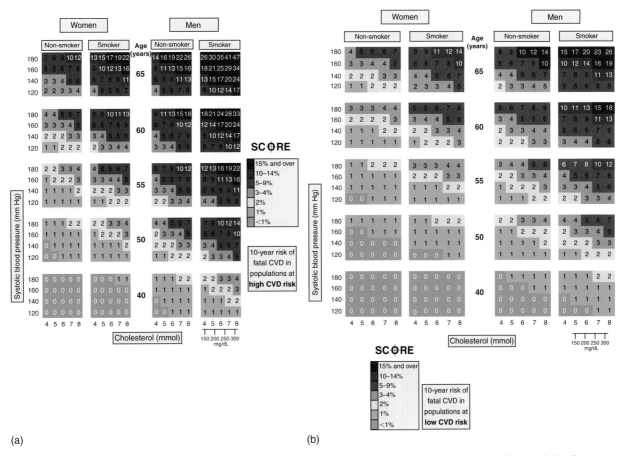

Figure 3.3 SCORE risk charts in (a) high-risk and (b) low-risk regions based on total cholesterol. *Source*: Reproduced with permission from Oxford University Press. Ref. 15.

Risk charts

Examples of the SCORE chart and a Framingham-based chart from the New Zealand guidelines are shown in Figures 3.3 and 3.4. To use the European SCORE charts to estimate risk, for example, find the table for gender, smoking status and age and the cell nearest to the person's blood pressure and total cholesterol. The person is categorised according to absolute 10-year risk for fatal CVD.

Computer-assisted algorithms

Several risk calculators are available online and can be downloaded from websites (Box 3.3); for example, HeartScore® is an electronic interactive tool based on the SCORE risk chart. It uses

the same risk factors and endpoints, but shows total risk in a bar chart and the distribution of modifiable risk factors in a pie chart.

Conclusion

This chapter has outlined the range of international recommendations on who to assess and how to estimate an individual's absolute cardiovascular risk to identify those patients at increased risk. While there are significant differences between guidelines, the main message of all guidelines is the same: multifactorial cardiovascular risk assessment is an essential prerequisite to effective and efficient management.

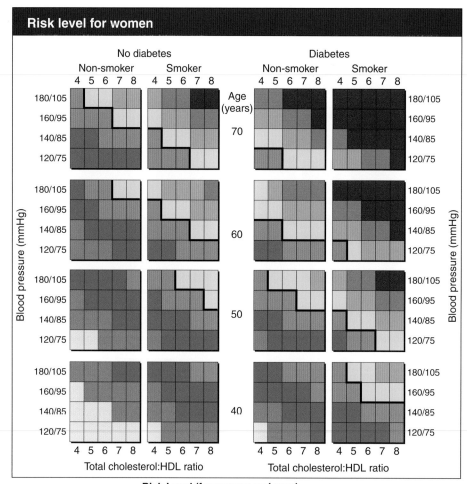

Risk level for women

Risk Level (for women and men)
5-year cardiovascular disease (CVD) risk (fatal and non-fatal)

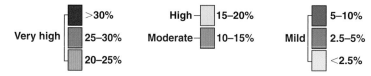

How to use the Charts
- Identify the chart relating to the person's sex, diabetic status, smoking history and age.
- Within the chart choose the cell nearest to the person's age, blood pressure (BP) and total cholesterol (TC) TC:HDL ratio. When the systolic and diastolic values fall in different risk levels, the higher category applies.
- For example, the lower left cell contains all non-smokers without diabetes who are less than 45 years and have a TC:HDL ratio of less than 4.5 and a BP of less than 130/80 mmHg. People who fall exactly on a threshold between cells are placed in the cell indicating higher risk.

(a)

Figure 3.4 Risk assessment charts from the New Zealand guidelines, based on the Framingham algorithm, (a) risk level in women and (b) risk level in men. *Source*: Reproduced with permission from New Zealand Guidelines Group. Ref. 19.

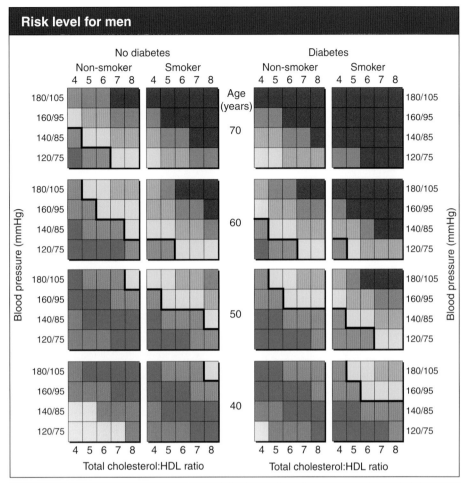

Based on the conservative estimate that each intervention: aspirin, BP treatment (lowering systolic BP by 10 mmHg) or lipid modification (lowering LDL-C by 20%) reduces cardiovascular risk by about 25% over 5 years.

Note: Cardiovascular events are defined as myocardial infarction, new angina, ischaemic stroke, transient ischaemic attack (TIA), peripheral vascular disease, congestive heart failure and cardiovascular-related death.

(b)   NNT = Number needed to treat.

Figure 3.4 (Continued).

Risk level 5-year CVD risk (fatal and non-fatal) (%)	Benefits: NNT for 5 years to prevent one event (CVD events prevented per 100 people treated for 5 years)		
	1 intervention (25% risk reduction)	2 interventions (45% risk reduction)	3 interventions (55% risk reduction)
30	13 (7.5 per 100)	7 (14 per 100)	6 (16 per 100)
20	20 (5 per 100)	11 (9 per 100)	9 (11 per 100)
15	27 (4 per 100)	15 (7 per 100)	12 (8 per 100)
10	40 (2.5 per 100)	22 (4.5 per 100)	18 (5.5 per 100)
5	80 (1.25 per 100)	44 (2.25 per 100)	36 (3 per 100)

Table 3.4 Risk categories according to different guidelines

Guideline	Outcomes: CHD/CVD; fatal/fatal and non-fatal events	Risk per year (%)		
		High	Moderate/ intermediate	Low
Australia	Fatal and non-fatal CVD	>3		
Canada	Fatal and non-fatal CHD risk	>2	1–2	<1
Europe	Fatal CVD risk	≥0.5		<0.5
New Zealand	Fatal and non-fatal CVD risk	>3	2–3	<2
USA	Fatal and non-fatal CHD risk	>2	1–2	<1
International	Fatal and non-fatal CHD risk	>2	1–2	<1

CVD: cardiovascular disease; CHD: coronary heart disease.

Box 3.3 Risk calculators available online

Framingham
- Adapted by NCEP ATP III
  - Risk calculator: http://hin.nhlbi.nih.gov/atpiii/calculator.asp?usertype=prof (online version)
  - Risk calculator: http://hin.nhlbi.nih.gov/atpiii/riskcalc.htm (downloadable version)
  - Risk calculator spreadsheet: http://www.nhlbi.nih.gov/guidelines/cholesterol/risk_tbl.htm
- Adapted by New Zealand Guidelines Group
  - Risk tables: http://www.nzgg.org.nz/guidelines/0035/CVD_Risk_Chart.pdf

SCORE
- SCORE risk charts: http://www.escardio.org/initiatives/prevention/SCORE+Risk+Charts.htm
- Heartscore®: http://www.escardio.org/knowledge/decision_tools/heartscore/Program+Download.htm

PROCAM
- Risk calculator: http://chdrisk.uni-muenster.de/calculator.php?iSprache=1&iVersion=1&iSiVersion=0
- Risk score: http://chdrisk.uni-muenster.de/risk.php?iSprache=1&iVersion=1&iSiVersion=0
- PROCAM Neuronal Network Analysis: http://chdrisk.uni-muenster.de/n_network.php?iSprache=1&iVersion=1&iSiVersion=0

UKPDS
- UKPDS Risk Engine: http://www.dtu.ox.ac.uk/index.html?maindoc=/ukpds/

Table 3.5 Study characteristics for data used in risk calculators

Study	Number	Age	Country	Ethnic group	Diabetes
FHS	2,590 men 2,983 women	30–74 years	United States	Mostly Caucasian	337
SCORE	88,080 men 117,098 women	19–80 years	11 European countries	European	Data not included
PROCAM	5,389 men	35–65 years	Germany	German	1,205 IFG, 406 diabetes
UKPDS	2,643 men 1,897 women	25–65 years	United Kingdom	Caucasian, Afro-Caribbean, Asian-Indian	All

FHS: Framingham Heart Study; SCORE: Systematic Coronary Risk Evaluation project; PROCAM: Prospective Cardiovascular Munster study; UKPDS: UK Prospective Diabetes Study; IFG: impaired fasting glycaemia.

References

1. Greenland P, Knoll MD, Stamler J, Neaton JD, Dyer AR, Garside DB et al. Major risk factors as antecedents of fatal and nonfatal coronary heart disease. *JAMA*. 2003; 290: 891–7.

2. Khot UN, Khot MB, Bajzer CT, Sapp SK, Ohman EM, Brener SJ et al. Prevalence of conventional risk factors in patients with coronary heart disease. *JAMA*. 2003; 290(7): 898–904.

3. Jackson R, Lawes CM, Bennett DA, Milne RJ, Rodgers A. Treatment with drugs to lower blood pressure and blood cholesterol based on an individual's absolute cardiovascular risk. *Lancet* 2005; 365: 434–41.

4. Genest J, Frohlich J, Fodor G, McPherson R. Recommendations for the management of dyslipidemia and the prevention of cardiovascular disease: 2003 update. *CMAJ*. 2003; 169: 921–4.

5. The assessment and management of cardiovascular risk. Available at http://www.nzgg.org.nz/index.cfm?fuseaction=fuseaction_10&fusesubaction=docs&documentid=22 (Accessed October 2007).

6. Donnelly R, Emslie-Smith AM, Gardner ID, et al. ABC of arterial and venous disease: Vascular complications of diabetes. *BMJ*. 2000; 320: 1062–6.

7. Haffner SM, Lehto S, Ronnemaa T et al. Mortality from coronary heart disease in subjects with type 2 diabetes and in nondiabetic subjects with and without prior myocardial infarction. *N Engl J Med*. 1998; 339: 229–34.

8. Third report of the National Cholesterol Education Program (NCEP) expert panel on detection, evaluation, and treatment of high blood cholesterol in adults (Adult Treatment Panel III) (2001). Expert panel on detection, evaluation, and treatment of high blood cholesterol in adults. *JAMA*. 2001; 285: 2486–97.

9. Grundy SM, Cleeman JI, Bairey CN et al. 2004 update – Implications of Recent Clinical Trials for the National Cholesterol Education Program Adult Treatment Panel III Guidelines. *Circulation*. 2004; 110: 227–39.

10. Graham I, Atar AE, Borch-Johsen K et al. European guidelines on cardiovascular disease prevention in clinical practice. *Eur J Cardiovasc Prev Rehabil*. 2007; 14(Suppl 2): S1–113.

11. Alberti KG, Zimmet P, Shaw J. IDF Epidemiology Task Force Consensus Group. The metabolic syndrome-a new worldwide definition. *Lancet*. 2005; 366: 1059–62.

12. Broedl UC, Geiss H-C, Parhofer KG. Comparison of current guidelines for primary prevention of coronary disease. *J Gen Intern Med*. 2003; 18: 190–5.

13. Haq IU, Ramsay LE, Jackson PR, Wallis EJ. Prediction of coronary risk for primary prevention of coronary heart disease: A comparison of methods. *QJM*. 1999; 92: 379–85.

14. Framingham Heart Study. Available at http://www.framinghamheart-study.org/about/index.html (Accessed October 2007).

15. Conroy RM, Pyorala K, Fitzgerald AP, Sans S, Menotti A, De Backer G et al. Estimation of ten-year risk of fatal cardiovascular disease in Europe: The SCORE project. *Eur Heart J*. 2003; 24(11): 987–1003.

16. Cullen P, Schulte H, Assmann G. The Münster Heart Study (PROCAM). Total mortality in middle-aged men is increased at low total and LDL cholesterol concentrations in smokers but not in non-smokers. *Circulation*. 1997; 96: 2128–36.

17. Stratton IM, Adler AI, Neil HA et al. Association of glycaemia with macrovascular and microvascular complications of type 2 diabetes (UKPDS 35): Prospective observational study. *BMJ*. 2000; 12; 321(7258): 405–12.

18. Turner RC, Millns H, Neil HA et al. Risk factors for coronary artery disease in non-insulin dependent diabetes mellitus: United Kingdom Prospective Diabetes Study (UKPDS 23). *BMJ*. 1998; 316(7134): 823–8.

19. UK Prospective Diabetes Study (UKPDS) Group. Intensive blood-glucose control with sulphonylureas or insulin compared with conventional treatment and risk of complications in patients with type 2 diabetes (UKPDS 33). *Lancet*. 1998; 352: 837–53.

20. UK Prospective Diabetes Study (UKPDS) Group. Effect of intensive blood-glucose control with metformin on complications in overweight patients with type 2 diabetes (UKPDS 34). *Lancet*. 1998; 352: 854–65.

21. Prevention of cardiovascular disease: An evidence-based clinical aid. *Med J Aust*. 2004; 181: F1–1.

22. International Atherosclerosis Society (IAS) (2003). Harmonized guidelines on prevention of atherosclerotic cardiovascular diseases. Available at http://www.athero.org/ (Accessed October 2007).

23. New Zealand Guidelines Group. *New Zealand Cardiovascular Guidelines Handbook: Developed for Primary Care Practitioners*. Wellington, New Zealand, 2003. www.nzgg.org.nz.

4

Moderate- to low-risk patients: management recommendations

J.I. Stewart[1], E. Washbrook[2] and A. Tonkin[3]

[1]University of Toronto, Ontario, Canada
[2]Future Forum Secretariat, London, UK
[3]Monash University, Australia

Introduction

Assessment of risk factors allows physicians to determine an individual's cardiovascular risk. The tools that are used to estimate risk are derived from prospective cohort studies and take into account the intensity of the range of important risk factors. 'High-risk' patients are generally defined as those whose 10-year risk of a coronary event is $\geq 20\%$, and include all individuals with established cardiovascular disease. Individuals at lower risk are classified as 'moderate- to low-risk' (e.g. 10-year risk $<20\%$) (Table 4.1). Although such individuals are asymptomatic, they are important targets for primary prevention of cardiovascular disease, particularly as the first clinical manifestation of coronary heart disease may be fatal. This article aims to provide practitioners with a concise guide to the management of moderate- to low-risk patients based on recommendations from some of the most up-to-date clinical practice guidelines for prevention of cardiovascular disease from different regions of the world (Box 4.1).[1-8] How to determine level of risk is discussed in this series in an article on 'Screening and identifying at-risk patients'.

Primary prevention of cardiovascular disease

Risk factors for cardiovascular disease may be present in childhood or early adulthood, but it may be decades before clinical disease manifests. However, early treatment to reduce risk factors may prevent onset of cardiovascular disease. To achieve this it is important to educate people identified as being at moderate to low risk about risk factors and lifestyle changes to help prevent them progressing to a higher risk status over time.

The concept of long-term risk can be used to emphasise the importance of reducing risk factors to young or middle-aged people who are at moderate to low risk. Figure 4.1 shows a portion of the SCORE risk chart that can be used to project long-term risk and illustrate how modifying risk factors can reduce or prevent the shift from low risk ($<5\%$ 10-year risk of fatal cardiovascular disease) to higher risk ($\geq 5\%$) over time.[10]

Treatment goals in moderate- to low-risk patients

The moderate- to low-risk category includes individuals at widely varying levels of risk (e.g. 10-year risk from 1 to 19%). Treatment goals and intensity should be related to the magnitude and immediacy of the cardiovascular risk. For example, individuals with a 10-year risk of 19% are at substantial short-term as well as long-term risk of a cardiovascular event. Treatment targets should therefore be fairly aggressive. In contrast, the short-term risk is obviously much lower for an individual with a 10-year risk of 1%, and therefore treatment does not need to be as intensive. The US National Cholesterol Education Program (NCEP) guidelines subdivide the moderate-to low-risk population into three categories (Table 4.2), and provide different recommendations for each group, but not all guidelines give detailed recommendations for patients with differing levels of risk in this category.[6,7] Clinical judgement is therefore important in determining appropriate treatment targets for individual patients.

Many people will have more than one cardiovascular risk factor such as cigarette smoking, dyslipidaemia or high blood pressure, and all relevant risk factors should be managed to reduce the long-term risk of cardiovascular events. Furthermore, a known risk factor may be just one component of the metabolic syndrome, which confers a considerably increased cardiovascular risk (see later articles in this series).

Cardiovascular Risk Management, Edited by R Hobbs and B Arroll
© 2009 Blackwell Publishing, ISBN: 9781405155755

Table 4.1 Risk categories according to different guidelines*

Guideline*	Risk period and endpoint	Risk (%)		
		High	Moderate/ intermediate	Low
Australia[a]	5-year CVD	>15[a]	–	–
Canada[b]	10-year CHD risk	>20	10–20	<10
Europe[c]	10-year fatal CVD risk	>5	–	<5
 **New Zealand**[a]	5-year cardiovascular risk	>15	10–15	<10
 **United States**[a]	10-year CHD risk	>20	1–20 2+ risk factors	<10 0–1 risk factor
International[a]	10-year CHD risk	>20	10–20	<10

[a] 10–15% 5-year CVD risk when either significant family history of premature CHD or metabolic is present.
[b] Risk assessment based on the Framingham algorithm.[9]
[c] Risk assessment based on the SCORE system.[10]
* See Box 4.1 for further details of the guidelines.
CVD: cardiovascular disease; CHD: coronary heart disease.

Box 4.1 Key regional guidelines for cardiovascular risk management

Australia
Position Statement on Lipid Management (2005)
http://www.heartfoundation.com.au/downloads/Lipids_HLCPosStatementFINAL_2005.pdf
• National Heart Foundation of Australia and Cardiac Society of Australia and New Zealand. *Heart Lung Circ.* 2005; 14: 275–91.
National Heart Foundation of Australia Hypertension Management Guide for Doctors (2004)
• *http://www.heartfoundation.com.au/downloads/hypertension_management_guide_2004.pdf*
Practical Implementation Taskforce for the Prevention of Cardiovascular Disease (2004)
• Prevention of cardiovascular disease: An evidence-based clinical aid. *Med J Aust.* 2004; 181: F1–14.
http://www.mja.com.au/public/issues/181_06_200904/ful10382_fm.html

Canada
Working Group on Hypercholesterolemia and Other Dyslipidemias (2003)
Genest J, Frohlich J, Fodor G, McPherson R. *CMAJ.* 2003; 169: 921–4.
http://www.cmaj.ca/cgi/content/full/169/9/921/DC1

Europe
Fourth Joint European Task Force (2007)
European Guidelines on Cardiovascular Disease Prevention in Clinical Practice
• Executive Summary: Graham I, Atar AE, Borch-Johsen K, et al. *Eur Heart J.* 2007; 28: 2375–414.
• Full text: Graham I, Atar AE, Borch-Johsen K, et al. *Eur J Cardiovasc Prev Rehabil.* 2007; 14(Suppl 2): S1–113.
http://www.escardio.org/knowledge/guidelines/CVD_Prevention_in_Clinical_Practice.htm

New Zealand
The New Zealand Guidelines Group (2003)
http://www.nzgg.org.nz/index.cfm?fuseaction=fuseaction_10&fusesubaction=docs&documentid=22

United States
National Cholesterol Education Program (2001, 2004)
http://www.nhlbi.nih.gov/guidelines/cholesterol/index.htm
• Expert panel on detection, evaluation, and treatment of high blood cholesterol in adults. *JAMA.* 2001; 285: 2486–97.
• Grundy SM, Cleeman JI, Bairey CN, et al. *Circulation.* 2004; 110: 227–39.

International
International Atherosclerosis Society (IAS) (2003)
http://www.athero.org/

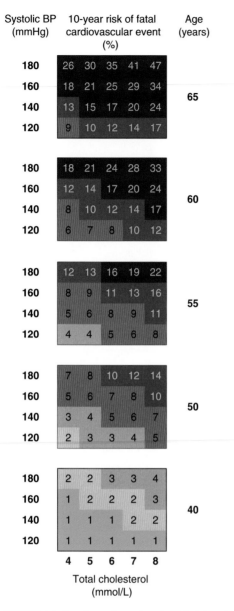

Systolic BP (mmHg) | 10-year risk of fatal cardiovascular event (%) | Age (years)

Figure 4.1 SCORE risk chart for male smokers in high-risk regions of Europe. The chart can be used to project an individual's current risk profile. For example, a male smoker at age 40 with 5 mmol/L total cholesterol and systolic blood pressure of 160 mmHg has a 10-year risk of a fatal cardiovascular event of 2%. However, if he reduces his total cholesterol or blood pressure (or stops smoking), his 10-year risk will fall to 1%. At the age of 65 the same risk profile will confer a 10-year risk of a fatal cardiovascular event of 21%. SCORE risk charts can be downloaded from the ESCardio website: http://www.escardio.org/ initiatives/prevention/SCORE+Risk+Charts.htm *Source*: Reproduced with permission from Oxford University Press. Ref. 10.

Recommended management strategies and treatment goals for moderate- to low-risk patients are summarised below. Lifestyle changes and therapies to achieve these goals are discussed later in this series.

Table 4.2 US NCEP LDL-C goals and cut points for therapeutic lifestyle changes (TLC) and drug therapy in moderate- to low-risk individuals

Risk category[a]		LDL-C goal	Initiate TLC	Consider drug therapy
Moderately high risk 2+ risk factors[b] (10-year risk 10–20%)		<3.3 mmol/L (<130 mg/dL) (optional goal <2.5 mmol/L [<100 mg/dL])	≥3.3 mmol/L (≥130 mg/dL)	≥3.3 mmol/L (≥130 mg/dL) (2.5–3.3 mmol/L [100–129 mg/dL]; consider drug options)
Moderate risk 2+ risk factors[b] (10-year risk <10%)		<3.3 mmol/L (<130 mg/dL)	≥3.3 mmol/L (≥130 mg/dL)	≥4.1 mmol/L (≥160 mg/dL)
Lower risk 0–1 risk factor[c]		<4.1 mmol/L (<160 mg/dL)	≥4.1 mmol/L (≥160 mg/dL)	≥4.9 mmol/L (≥190 mg/dL) (4.1–4.8 mmol/L [160–189 mg/dL]: LDL-lowering drug optional)

[a] According to the NCEP guidelines, individuals are assigned to three risk categories through a combination of risk factor assessment and the Framingham algorithm.
[b] Risk factors include cigarette smoking, hypertension (BP >140/90 mmHg or on antihypertensive medication), low HDL-C (<1 mmol/L [<40 mg/dL]), family history of premature coronary heart disease (coronary heart disease in male first-degree relative <55 years of age; coronary heart disease in female first-degree relative <65 years of age) and age (men >45 years; women >55 years).
[c] Almost all people with zero or one risk factor have a 10-year risk <10%, and 10-year risk assessment in people with zero or one risk factor is thus not necessary.

Stop cigarette smoking

Cigarette smoking can substantially increase cardiovascular risk and stopping smoking is an important target for reducing risk. Smoking cessation is recommended for individuals at all levels of cardiovascular risk by most guidelines under consideration. The USA and Canadian guidelines recognise smoking as a major risk factor, without explicitly recommending smoking cessation.[3,6,7]

Improve lipid levels

Treatment of dyslipidaemia is fundamental to cardiovascular disease prevention in all at-risk populations. Reducing low-density lipoprotein (LDL-C) is the most frequently recommended treatment goal for individuals at moderate to low risk (Table 4.3). Reduction of total cholesterol or total cholesterol:HDL-C ratio is also recommended by some guidelines as additional or alternative targets. Even in individuals with low HDL-C and high triglyceride levels, reducing LDL-C is recommended as

Table 4.3 Lipid goals in moderate- to low-risk individuals (e.g. 10-year risk of a coronary event <20%) included in different guidelines

Guideline	Cut point for initiation of lipid-modifying therapy	Goal		
		LDL-C (mmol/L)	TC (mmol/L)	TC:HDL-C ratio
Australia	TC: 8.0 mmol/L	4	4	4
Canada	None stated	<3.5 or 4.5[a]	–	<5.0 or 6.0[a]
Europe	None stated	<3.0	<5.0	–
New Zealand	TC: 8.0 mmol/L TC:HDL-C ratio: 8.0	Determine appropriate goals for each patient to reduce 5-year CVD risk using risk charts		
United States	LDL-C: 3.3–4.9 mmol/L[a]	<3.3 or 4.1[a]	–	–
International	LDL-C: 3.4–4.9 mmol/L[a,b]	<3.4 or 4.1[a]	–	–

[a]Goal/cut point depends on disease status/level of risk (see Table 4.1 for breakdown of USA goals/cut points).
[b]Use of drugs should depend on national healthcare policy.
NB. Attempts should also be made to increase HDL-C and lower triglyceride levels in appropriate patients.
CVD: cardiovascular disease; LDL-C: low-density lipoprotein cholesterol; TC: total cholesterol; HDL-C: high-density lipoprotein cholesterol.

Table 4.4 Blood pressure goals in moderate- to low-risk individuals (10-year risk of a coronary event <20%) included in different guidelines

Guideline	Cut point for initiating therapy (mmHg)	Blood pressure goal (mmHg)
Australia	Patients <65 years: >180/105[a] Patients >65 years: >160/100[a]	<140/90 unless <65 years, diabetes, renal insufficiency and/or proteinuria
Canada	–	–
Europe	≥180/110	<140/90
New Zealand	>170/100 115/70–170/100 dependent on risk level	<140/85[b]
United States	–	–
International	–	<140/90

[a]Recommendations depend on associated clinical conditions, whether target organ damage or indigenous person.
[b]Lower lipid and blood pressure targets may be chosen, and should be individualised according to level of risk as determined using a risk chart.

the primary goal. However, there is general agreement that attempts should be made to modify HDL-C and triglyceride levels in all individuals in whom these lipids are not optimal.

In the moderate- to low-risk population, treatment recommendations for dyslipidaemia are based primarily on lifestyle modification, particularly diet. The guidelines differ in their recommendations regarding initiating lipid-lowering drugs. For example, the US NCEP guidelines cite specific cut points for the initiation of lipid-lowering agents (Table 4.1), while the European guidelines do not discuss the use of drugs in this population.[4,6,7] To some extent, these differences reflect variations among countries and regions in healthcare budgets and priorities.

Reduce high blood pressure

The recommended blood pressure goals for individuals at moderate- to low-risk of cardiovascular disease are less strict than those recommended for high-risk patients (Table 4.4). This reflects the basic tenet that intensity of treatment should be related to individual risk. It is generally accepted that initial attempts to reduce blood pressure should be based on therapeutic changes in lifestyle (e.g. weight reduction, dietary modification including sodium and alcohol restriction, increase in physical activity). If this is ineffective, or if blood pressure is considerably elevated, antihypertensive medication should be introduced. The guidelines vary in their recommendations regarding the level at which antihypertensive medication should be introduced (Table 4.4).

Reduce bodyweight

Weight reduction is an important goal in all overweight individuals. Bodyweight can be quantified by calculating body mass index (BMI = weight [kg]/height [m^2]). BMI values of 18.5–25 kg/m^2 are regarded as normal, but may vary according to ethnic group (e.g. the upper threshold for South East Asians may be lower).[11] In individuals whose BMI exceeds this range, increasing bodyweight is associated with a continuous rise

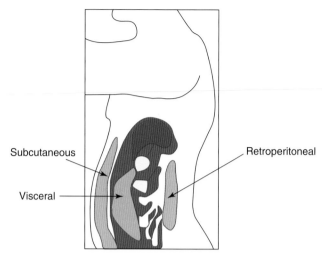

Figure 4.2 Location of fat in people with abdominal obesity. Fat located in the abdominal region is associated with greater cardiovascular risk than that in peripheral regions. Abdominal fat has three components: visceral, retroperitoneal and subcutaneous. Waist or abdominal circumference, as well as BMI, should be measured for the assessment of obesity, and as a guide to weight loss.

Table 4.5 US NCEP LDL-C recommendations for therapeutic dietary goals to reduce LDL-C

Dietary component	Sources	Recommendation
Components that increase LDL-C		
Saturated fatty acids	High-fat dairy products and meat, tropical oils (e.g. coconut), baked products	Should make up <7% of total calorie intake
Dietary cholesterol	Eggs, meat, dairy, poultry, shellfish	<200 mg/day
Components that reduce LDL-C		
Monosaturated fats	Plant oils, nuts	Up to 20% total calorie intake
Polyunsaturated fats	Liquid vegetable oils, semi-liquid margarines	Up to 10% total calorie intake
Viscous (soluble) fibre	Oats, barley, pectin-rich fruit, beans	5–10 g/day
Plant stanol/sterol esters	Soybean, tall pine-tree oils, commercial margarines	2 g/day

in the risk of cardiovascular risk factors and coronary heart disease. Cardiovascular risk is most closely related to abdominal obesity (Figure 4.2), which can be estimated by measuring waist circumference. Indeed, the presence of excess fat in the abdomen, out of proportion to total body fat, is an independent predictor of cardiovascular risk factors and morbidity. Waist-to-hip ratio (WHR) is another measurement that can indicate the presence of excess fat in the abdomen. In men a WHR of >0.95 and in women a WHR of >0.80 indicates a health risk.

All individuals who are overweight (BMI $\geqslant$25 kg/m^2) or obese (BMI $\geqslant$30 kg/m^2), or who have increased waist circumference (>102 cm in men, >88 cm in women) should aim to reduce bodyweight/waist circumference to within the normal range. Achievement of these goals is based primarily on dietary modification and increased physical activity. Behavioural therapy may be required to maintain long-term control of bodyweight.[12]

Improve diet

Adoption of a cardioprotective diet is recommended for all individuals. The main emphasis is on low-fat dietary constituents. In particular, cholesterol intake and the percentage of saturated fat and trans-fatty acids should be minimised. Examples of dietary goals for reducing LDL-C levels from the US NCEP guidelines are summarised in Table 4.5.[6,7] In addition to controlling the intake of atherogenic dietary constituents, efforts should be made to increase consumption of cardioprotective foods such as fruits and vegetables and omega-3 fatty acids (available particularly in oily fish). For overweight and obese individuals, energy intake should be reduced by

---

Box 4.2 Dietary strategies to reduce postprandial hyperglycaemia

Each day:

- Consume $\geqslant$40 g of dietary fibre
- Distribute carbohydrate intake evenly throughout the day

At each meal:

- Include high-fibre foods with a low-to-moderate glycaemic index
- Avoid a large volume of carbohydrate-rich food.

500–1,000 kcal/day with the initial aim of reducing bodyweight by 10% within 6 months.

Reduce hyperglycaemia/insulin resistance

Many individuals display a level of insulin resistance or impaired glucose tolerance that increases their risk of atherosclerotic disease but that is not sufficiently severe to merit a diagnosis of Type 2 diabetes (which would consign them to the 'high-risk' category).

Reduction of insulin resistance is based on weight reduction and increased physical activity, both of which should be encouraged and supported. However, as emphasised by the New Zealand NZGG guidelines, a number of dietary strategies may help to control postprandial hyperglycaemia (Box 4.2).[5]

Box 4.3 Ethnic groups considered in the US, Australian and New Zealand guidelines

NCEP guidelines

- Despite some differences in baseline risk for these populations vs white Americans, it is recommended that the guidelines are appropriate for all groups:
  - **African Americans** (special attention should be paid to some features of risk management)
  - **Hispanic American**
  - **Native Americans**
  - **Asian and Pacific Islanders**
  - **South Asians** (special attention should be given to detection of CHD risk factors)

National heart Foundation of Australia

- **Aboriginal and Torres Strait Islander people** – more prevalent and much higher age-standardised mortality from CVD
  - Recommend screening for lipid levels commence at 18 years then annually
  - Caution advised in direct use of usual absolute risk equations as derived from Framingham

NZGG guidelines

- **Māoris, Pacific Islander and Indian Subcontinent people**
  - more prevalent and earlier occurrence of CVD and cardiovascular death than in New Zealanders of European descent
  - Cardiovascular risk assessment should begin 10 years earlier
  - Māori Cardiovascular Action Plan initiated – prioritise Māori cardiovascular health.

The use of insulin-sensitising agents for non-diabetic individuals is not currently recommended by any of the guidelines.

Management of population subgroups

It is well recognised that the risk of cardiovascular disease is affected by factors such as gender and ethnic background. For example, the onset of coronary heart disease is delayed on average by about 10 years in women compared with men, and therefore the recommended age at which routine screening is initiated is earlier in men than women. The New Zealand NZGG and US NCEP guidelines consider management of certain ethnic groups (Box 4.3).[5–7] It is important that healthcare providers are aware of both the risk factors and social differences of ethnic populations when assessing risk for cardiovascular disease and implementing prevention strategies. However, once an individual's cardiovascular risk has been established, recommended treatment goals are not influenced by either gender or ethnicity.

Conclusions

For individuals with a moderate to low risk of cardiovascular disease, prevention of cardiovascular events is an important target, with treatment goals and intensity related to the magnitude and immediacy of the individual's total cardiovascular risk. Since the moderate- to low-risk category includes individuals at widely varying levels of risk, clinical judgement is of over-riding importance in managing this heterogeneous group of individuals.

Intervention should be centred around therapeutic changes in lifestyle. In general, pharmaceutical agents are used fairly sparingly in this group, and are reserved for cases in which lifestyle modification has failed to achieve the desired degree of risk reduction.

References

1. National Heart Foundation of Australia and Cardiac Society of Australia and New Zealand. *Heart, Lung Circ.* 2005; 14: 275–91.
2. Prevention of cardiovascular disease: An evidence-based clinical aid. *Med J Aust.* 2004; 181: F1–14.
3. Genest J, Frohlich J, Fodor G, McPherson R. Recommendations for the management of dyslipidemia and the prevention of cardiovascular disease: 2003 update. *CMAJ.* 2003; 169: 921–4.
4. Graham I, Atar AE, Borch-Johsen K et al. European guidelines on cardiovascular disease prevention in clinical practice. *Eur J Cardiovasc Prev Rehabil.* 2007; 14(Suppl 2): S1–113.
5. The assessment and management of cardiovascular risk. Available at http://www.nzgg.org.nz/index.cfm?fuseaction=fuseaction_10&fusesubaction=docs&documentid=22 (Accessed October 2007).
6. Third report of the National Cholesterol Education Program (NCEP) expert panel on detection, evaluation, and treatment of high blood cholesterol in adults (Adult Treatment Panel III) (2001). Expert Panel on Detection, Evaluation, and Treatment of High Blood Cholesterol in Adults. *JAMA.* 2001; 285: 2486–97.
7. Grundy SM, Cleeman JI, Bairey CN et al. Implications of Recent Clinical Trials for the National Cholesterol Education Program Adult Treatment Panel III Guidelines – 2004 update. *Circulation.* 2004; 110: 227–39.
8. International Atherosclerosis Society (IAS) (2003). Harmonized guidelines on prevention of atherosclerotic cardiovascular diseases. Available at http://www.athero.org/ (Accessed October 2007).
9. Framingham Heart Study. Available at http://www.framinghamheartstudy.org/about/index.html. (Accessed October 2007).
10. Conroy RM, Pyorala K, Fitzgerald AP, Sans S, Menotti A, De Backer G et al. Estimation of ten-year risk of fatal cardiovascular disease in Europe: The SCORE project. *Eur Heart J.* 2003; 24(11): 987–1003.
11. Razak F et al. Defining obesity cut points in a multiethnic population. *Circulation.* 2007; 115(16): 2111–8.
12. Guidelines on the management of adult obesity and overweight in primary care. National Obesity Forum. Available at: http://nationalobesityforum.org.uk/images/stories/W_M_guidelines/NOF_Adult_Guildelines_Feb_06.pdf (Accessed October 2007).

5

High-risk patients: management recommendations

D. Duhot,[1] E. McGregor[2] and C. Packard[3]

[1] Société Française de Médecine Générale, Issy les Moulineaux, France
[2] The Future Forum Secretariat, London, UK
[3] Department of Pathological Biochemistry, Glasgow Royal Infirmary, Alexandra Parade, Glasgow, UK

Introduction

For people identified as being at risk of cardiovascular disease (CVD), the degree or intensity of intervention is dictated by the predicted likelihood of a future coronary event. Assessment of cardiovascular risk factors is therefore essential so that individuals can be stratified as accurately as possible into 'very high', 'high' or 'moderate-to-low' risk categories (see chapter on 'Screening and identifying at-risk patients' in this book).

The high-risk category (Box 5.1) includes all those with established cardiovascular, cerebrovascular or peripheral vascular disease, or with diabetes; a subset of these regarded as 'very high' risk are targeted for more aggressive intervention (Box 5.2). Appropriate screening can identify asymptomatic individuals who are considered also to be at high risk due to the presence of multiple risk factors. Although there is some variation between guidelines in the definition of 'high cardiovascular risk', this term usually refers to patients whose 10-year risk of an atherosclerotic coronary event (e.g. myocardial infarction) is $\geqslant 20\%$ (see chapter in book – Screening and identifying at-risk patients).

This chapter aims to provide practitioners with a concise guide to the management of high-risk patients based on recommendations from six of the most up-to-date clinical practice guidelines for prevention of CVD (Box 5.3).[1-7] We refer non-English speakers to the French Health Products Safety Agency and the Spanish local guidelines.[8,9]

Treatment goals in high-risk patients

Once a patient's high-risk status has been established, it is important to address all risk factors amenable to intervention including cigarette smoking, serum lipid levels, hypertension,

Cardiovascular Risk Management, Edited by R Hobbs and B Arroll
© 2009 Blackwell Publishing, ISBN: 9781405155755

hyperglycaemia/insulin resistance, excess body weight and thrombotic risk.[10] Many of these are improved by lifestyle changes (Box 5.4) but for the majority of high-risk individuals drug therapy will also be needed and should be introduced without undue delay.

Summarised below are the recommended treatment goals in high-risk patients.

Stop cigarette smoking

Cigarette smoking, one of the strongest risk factors for atherosclerotic disease, has a dose-dependent effect on cardiovascular risk. As recommended by most guidelines (Table 5.1), all patients who smoke should be encouraged strongly and assisted actively to stop, since a reduction in risk may be observed within a few months of smoking cessation. Nicotine replacement therapy (NRT) in combination with simple or intensive behavioural support is an effective strategy. In practice, smoking cessation can be achieved in up to 19% of smoking patients. In one study, smoking cessation was achieved in 24.5% of patients using NRT after 12 weeks (compared with 14.2% on placebo) and 10.8% after 12 months (compared with 7.7% on placebo).[11]

Improve lipid levels

The strong, positive association between total serum cholesterol levels and atherosclerotic disease was recognised over 50 years ago. Cholesterol in the circulation is carried in low-density lipoprotein (LDL-C), which is atherogenic, and high-density lipoprotein cholesterol (HDL-C), which protects against atherosclerosis.

LDL-C and total cholesterol

Although total cholesterol is still widely targeted as a goal in preventative strategies, there is agreement among the guidelines that LDL-C should be the primary lipid target in almost all at-risk individuals. For those at high risk, LDL-C should be lowered to <2.5 mmol/L (Table 5.2). US guidelines recommend

Box 5.1 High-risk patients (conversion of units in Box 5.6)

Patients in the 'high-risk' category have

- Coronary heart disease and stroke
- Peripheral arterial disease
- Abdominal aortic aneurysm
- Symptomatic carotid artery disease (transient ischaemic attack)

OR

- Diabetes

OR

- Presence of multiple risk factors to give predicted 10 year CHD risk >20%
  These factors include:
  - Cigarette smoking or cessation less than 3 years
  - High LDL-C (≥4.1 mmol/L) or total cholesterol (≥6.2 mmol/L)[a]
  - Low HDL-C (<1 mmol/L)
  - Hypertension (blood pressure ≥140/90 mmHg or on antihypertensive medication)
  - History of premature coronary heart disease in a first-degree relative (i.e. event in a male <55 years or female <65 years)

Source: Adapted from Ref. 1. Other guidelines (see Box 5.4) specify LDL-C and total cholesterol cutoffs of 6.0 and 8.0 mmol/L, respectively. Risk calculation tools are available at:

European risk calculator for the prediction and management of the risk of heart attack and stroke in Europe: http://www.escardio.org/knowledge/decision_tools/heartscore/

General predictive tool for calculating primary risk analysis over 10 years (not based on country of origin): http://www.bhsoc.org/riskcalc/riskcalculator.exe

---

Box 5.2 Very high-risk patients (conversion of units in Box 5.6)

- Patients in the 'very high' risk category have established CVD plus
  - The presence of multiple major risk factors (see Box 5.1) or diabetes
  - Severe and poorly controlled risk factors (especially cigarette smoking) (see Box 5.1)
  - Multiple features of the metabolic syndrome (see Box 5.5)
  - Acute coronary syndrome
- Treatment is aggressive with institution of diet and lifestyle modification and immediate commencement of statin therapy
- Goal of lipid lowering treatment is LDL-C <1.8 mmol/L (<70 mg/dL)

Source: Adapted from Ref. 2.

Box 5.3 Regional and national guidelines for prevention of CVD

Australia	**Practical Implementation Taskforce for the Prevention of Cardiovascular Disease (2004)** Prevention of cardiovascular disease: An evidence-based clinical aid. *Med J Aust.* 2004; 181: F1–14. http://www.mja.com.au/public/issues/181_06_200904/ful10382_fm.html
Canada	**Working Group on Hypercholesterolemia and Other Dyslipidemias (2003)** Genest J, Frohlich J, Fodor G, McPherson R. Recommendations for the management of dyslipidemia and the prevention of cardiovascular disease: 2003 update. *CMAJ.* 2003; 169: 921–4. http://www.cmaj.ca/cgi/content/full/169/9/921/DC1
Europe	**Fourth Joint European Task Force (2007)** Executive Summary: Graham I, Atar AE, Borch-Johsen K et al. European guidelines on cardiovascular disease prevention in clinical practice. *Eur Heart J.* 2007; 28: 2375–414. Full text: Graham I, Atar AE, Borch-Johsen K et al. European guidelines on cardiovascular disease prevention in clinical practice. *Eur J Cardiovasc Prev Rehabil.* 2007; 14(Suppl 2): S1–113. http://www.escardio.org/knowledge/guidelines/CVD_Prevention_in_Clinical_Practice.htm
New Zealand	**The New Zealand Guidelines Group (2003)** The assessment and management of cardiovascular risk. http://www.nzgg.org.nz/index.cfm?fuseaction=fuseaction_10&fusesubaction=docs&documentid=22
United States 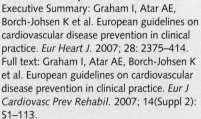	**National Cholesterol Education Program (2001, 2004)** Third report of the National Cholesterol Education Program (NCEP) expert panel on detection, evaluation, and treatment of high blood cholesterol in adults (Adult Treatment Panel III) (2001). Expert panel on detection, evaluation, and treatment of high blood cholesterol in adults. *JAMA.* 2001; 285: 2486–97. Grundy SM, Cleeman JI, Bairey CN et al. Implications of recent clinical trials for the national cholesterol education program adult treatment panel III guidelines – 2004 update. *Circulation.* 2004; 110: 227–39. http://www.nhlbi.nih.gov/guidelines/cholesterol/index.htm
International	**International Atherosclerosis Society (IAS) (2003)** Harmonized guidelines on prevention of atherosclerotic cardiovascular diseases. http://www.athero.org/

that patients at very high risk would benefit from a lower LDL-C goal (<1.8–2.0 mmol/L). In addition to an absolute target level, some guidelines recommend that LDL-C be reduced by at least 30% and it is believed that there is a linear relationship between fall in LDL-C and reduction in risk.

HDL-C and triglycerides

Some guidelines recommend total cholesterol: HDL-C ratio as an alternative target benchmark for intervention (Table 5.2). Low levels of HDL-C and elevated triglyceride levels are both associated with increased cardiovascular risk, and are frequently present in individuals with Type 2 diabetes or the metabolic syndrome (Box 5.5).[12] Most of the guidelines regard a triglyceride level <1.7 mmol/L as desirable. Target HDL-C levels are rarely stated, but there is widespread agreement that cardiovascular risk is increased when HDL-C <1.0 mmol/L in men and <1.3 mmol/L in women (Box 5.6).

Box 5.4 Lifestyle changes that reduce cardiovascular risk

- Smoking cessation
- Dietary modification (see Table 5.5)
- Achievement of ideal bodyweight (BMI <25 kg/m²; see Figure 5.1)
- Increased physical activity

Reduce high blood pressure

Cardiovascular risk rises continuously as the degree of hypertension increases. Effort should be made to reduce elevated blood pressure by changes in lifestyle, which, if necessary, should be combined with antihypertensive medication. Target systolic pressures of 130–140 mmHg and diastolic pressures of 85–90 mmHg are recommended by three of the six practice guidelines (Table 5.3). A lower target level (130/80 mmHg) is appropriate for people with diabetes and CHD. Many studies have confirmed that multiple therapies will usually be necessary to achieve these blood pressure targets, and several guidelines highlight this strategy.

Reduce hyperglycaemia/insulin resistance

The incidence of macrovascular disease in patients with diabetes may be related to blood glucose control. As a result, three of the six practice guidelines recommend that hyperglycaemia should be controlled to maintain $HbA_{1c} \leq 6$ or $\leq 7\%$ (Table 5.4).

Reduce bodyweight

Weight reduction is an important goal in overweight or obese high-risk individuals. Bodyweight is most readily quantified as body mass index (BMI; Figure 5.1).[13] Individuals with BMI values ≥ 25 kg/m² should receive counselling and help in achieving bodyweight reduction. Cardiovascular risk is also influenced by the regional distribution of body fat, and abdominal fat is particularly detrimental. Patients with abdominal obesity (commonly defined as a waist circumference >102 cm

---

Table 5.1 Recommended management of risk factors in high-risk individuals

	Guideline (see Box 5.3 for full reference)					
	Australia	Canada	Europe	New Zealand	United States	International
Goal or treatment recommended?						
Smoking cessation	✓	–	✓	✓	–	✓
Lifestyle change[a]	✓	✓	✓	✓	✓[b]	✓
Dyslipidaemia	✓	✓	✓	✓	✓	✓
Blood pressure	✓[c]	–	✓	✓	–	✓
Antiplatelet therapy	✓	–	✓	✓	–	✓
Control of hyperglycaemia (diabetes patients)	–	–	✓	✓	–	✓

Note: 10-year risk of a cardiovascular event ≥20%.
[a]Prudent diet, achievement of optimal bodyweight, increased physical activity.
[b]Optional if low-density lipoprotein cholesterol <2.6 mmol/L.
[c]Recommended in selected patient subgroups only.
The use of beta-blockers, angiotensin converting enzyme inhibitors and anticoagulants is recommended by most guidelines, where appropriate.

Table 5.2 Lipid goals in high-risk individuals (conversion of units in Box 5.6)

Guideline	Threshold for initiating treatment[a]	Goal[b]		
		LDL-C (mmol/L)	TC (mmol/L)	TC: HDL-C ratio
Australia	TC: 3.5/5.0 mmol/L[c]	–	<3.5/5.0[c]	–
Canada	Treatment recommended in all patients	<2.5	–	<4.0
Europe	TC: 5.0 mmol/L LDL-C: 3.0 mmol/L	<2.5	<4.5	–
New Zealand	TC: 8.0 mmol/L TC:HDL-C: 8.0	<2.0/2.5[c]	<3.5/4.0[c]	<4.5
United States	LDL-C: 2.6 mmol/L (optional if LDL-C< 2.6 mmol/L)	↓ by 30–40% and to <1.8/2.6[c]	–	–
International	Treatment recommended in all patients	↓ by 30% and to <2.6	–	–

[a]Threshold for initiation of lipid-modifying drugs.
[b]Attempts should also be made to increase HDL-C and lower triglyceride levels in appropriate patients.
[c]Goal/cutpoint depends on disease status/level of risk.

Box 5.5 Features of the metabolic syndrome (conversion of units in Box 5.6)

- Metabolic syndrome is diagnosed when there is central obesity as assessed by waist circumference
  - 94 cm in European men, >80 cm in European women
  - >90 cm in South Asian men, >80 cm in South Asian women
- Plus two of the following:
  - Triglycerides ≥1.7 mmol/L (150 mg/dL)
  - HDL-C <1.03 mmol/L in men (<40 mg/dL in men)
  - Blood pressure ≥130/85 mmHg or an antihypertensive Px
  - Glucose ≥5.6 mmol/L (100 mg/dL) or known diabetic

The IDF definition of the metabolic syndrome.
For the Third Report of the National Cholesterol Education Program (2001), the International Atherosclerosis Society Harmonized guidelines (2003), see Box 5.3.

Box 5.6 Conversion coefficients

- **Cholesterol**
  - g/L × 2.58 = mmol/L
  - mg/dL × 0.258 = mmol/L
  - mmol/L × 0.387 = g/L
  - mmol/L × 38.7 = mg/dL
- **Triglycerides**
  - g/L × 1.14 = mmol/L
  - mg/dL × 0.0114 = mmol/L
  - mmol/L × 0.875 = g/L
  - mmol/L × 87.5 = mg/dL

physical activity. In high-risk patients, the recommended level of physical exertion should be based on the results of a comprehensive clinical evaluation. Inclusion of an exercise test in this evaluation is discretionary. Achieving a 5% reduction in body weight is a good first step.

Improve diet

For patients at high risk of CVD, dietary modification has two main aims: (i) to lower LDL-C; (ii) to allow the patient to achieve

in American men, >88 cm in American women) should be encouraged to lose weight, regardless of BMI.

Weight loss is difficult to achieve and maintain, but must involve a combination of dietary modification and increased

Table 5.3 Blood pressure goals in high-risk individuals

Guideline		Blood pressure goal (mmHg)
	Australia	<140/90 or <130/85 [a,b]
	Canada	–
	Europe	<140/90 or <130/80 [a]
	New Zealand	<140/85 or <130/80[a,c,d]
	United States	–
	International	<130/85

The lower goal is recommended for patients with
[a]Diabetes.
[b]Renal disease.
[c]Clinical CVD.
[d]Aggressive management of blood pressure is recommended for patients with diabetes and concomitant renal disease.

Table 5.4 HbA$_{1c}$ goals in individuals with diabetes

Guideline		HbA$_{1c}$ (%)
	Australia	–
	Canada	–
	Europe	≤6.1
	New Zealand	≤7
	United States	–
	International	≤7

an optimal bodyweight. Table 5.5 summarises the core dietary recommendations made by the guidelines.[1–7,14] In addition to providing detailed recommendations on lipid intake, the guidelines recommend minimum daily intakes of dietary constituents believed to provide protection against CVD such as omega-3 fatty acids and fruits and vegetables.

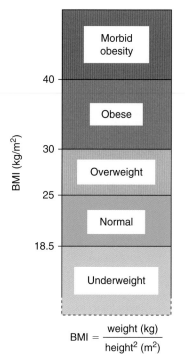

$$BMI = \frac{weight~(kg)}{height^2~(m^2)}$$

Figure 5.1 Body mass index.* *BMI ranges recommended by the US National Heart Lung and Blood Institute (NHLBI). Recommended BMI ranges may vary from country to country. If weight reduction is necessary, energy intake should be reduced by 500–1,000 kcal/day with the initial aim of reducing bodyweight by 10% within 6 months. A BMI calculator that uses both metric and imperial measurements is available on the US NHLBI website: http://nhlbisupport.com/bmi/bmicalc.htm

Table 5.5 Major dietary requirements for individuals at high cardiovascular risk

Nutrient	Recommended intake
Total calories	Adjust to achieve/maintain desirable bodyweight (BMI <25 kg/m^2)
Total fat	25–35% of total calories
Saturated fat and trans-fatty acids	<7% of total calories
Polyunsaturated fat	≤10% of total calories
Monounsaturated fat	≤20% of total calories
Cholesterol	<200 mg/day
Carbohydrate	50–60% of total calories
Protein	Approximately 15% of total calories
Fibre	20–30 g/day
Omega-3 fatty acids	≥1% of total calories or up to 1 g/day
Fruit and vegetables	≥5 servings/day
Alcohol	≤20–30 g ethanol/day (men), ≤10–20 g/ day (women)

Practical dietary guidelines for patients that provide recommendations similar to those above are available at the American Heart Association website: http://www.americanheart.org/presenter.jhtml?identifier=851

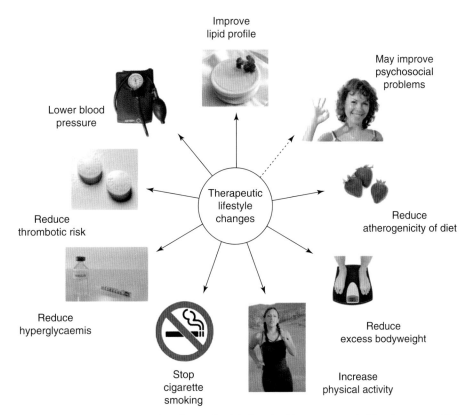

Figure 5.2 Therapeutic lifestyle changes lead to reduced cardiovascular risk. Sustained improvements in lifestyle are more likely to occur if patient care includes explicit instructions, extensive education, behavioural counselling and frequent follow-up.

Reduce thrombotic risk

With few exceptions, acute cardiovascular events are caused by formation of an intra-arterial thrombus. Antiplatelet therapy (e.g. aspirin at a dose of between 75 and 150 mg daily) is therefore widely recommended for routine use in all patients at risk of atherothrombosis (Table 5.1). Anticoagulants may also be employed.

Management of population subgroups

The recommendations discussed above apply to all high-risk individuals. However, in some cases, special consideration may be required in view of the patient's age or ethnic origin.

Elderly subjects

Historically, healthcare policy-makers and physicians have not pursued aggressive modification of cardiovascular risk factors in the elderly. However, recent clinical trials have shown conclusively that LDL-lowering leads to substantial reductions in cardiovascular risk in high-risk elderly individuals. These findings have led three of the six guidelines to emphasise that elderly patients should not be denied treatment of dyslipidaemia on the basis of age alone. After the age of 80 years the treatment of

hypercholesterolaemia depends on the extent of cardiovascular risk factors, the general health of the patient (i.e. are they suffering from an illness other than CVD that may decrease their life expectancy) and general tolerance to medication.

Ethnic groups

A patient's ethnic background may also require consideration, since it is well established that the incidence of CVD and certain risk factors differs among populations. Some guidelines use ethnicity or country of origin as a major factor in determining total cardiovascular risk, for example in the United Kingdom, standardised mortality rates for CHD are notably increased among south Asian immigrants and this ethnic background is counted as an independent risk factor.[15] Others adjust the baseline risk according to ethnicity (New Zealand guidelines with Maori, Pacific and Indian subcontinent).[6] However, none of the guidelines recommend modifying treatment goals on the basis of ethnic origin.

Putting risk factor reduction into practice

Optimal medical management of high-risk patients requires a holistic approach to care. This should lead to improvements in multiple risk factors, including dyslipidaemia, hypertension, thrombotic state and hyperglycaemia. For a comprehensive risk reduction strategy, patient education and motivation are vital, and communication with the patient is fundamental to successful implementation. Techniques that encourage patient compliance will be discussed later in this book.

Treatment strategies

Many risk factors can be modified by lifestyle changes, which form the basis of risk reduction for all patients (Figure 5.2). However, in high-risk patients adequate improvement in risk profile is rarely achieved using non-pharmacological management alone and these patients usually require treatment with lipid-modifying and antihypertensive drugs. Diabetic patients may also require antihyperglycaemic medication. Treatment strategies, including lifestyle changes, to modify cardiovascular risk factors to target levels will be discussed later in this book.

Patient well-being

The cardiovascular health of high-risk patients may be affected by psychosocial factors including depression and social isolation in addition to physical factors. As emphasised by the European guidelines, physicians play an important role in ensuring such patients receive appropriate help.

Conclusion

Management of the high-risk cardiovascular patient requires simultaneous, aggressive reduction of multiple risk factors to recommended goals, and therefore commitment to the management regimen is of fundamental importance.

Therapeutic changes in lifestyle, which are integral to patient management, can lead to substantial risk reduction. In addition, in high-risk patients, immediate institution of pharmacological (lipid-lowering, antihypertensive and antiplatelet where appropriate) therapy is usually recommended to enable risk reduction targets to be achieved.

Patient perceptions and knowledge regarding level of cardiovascular risk differ from those of care providers and may impede risk modification. This has implications for health education and should be considered when providing tailored care for patients.[16]

References

1. Third report of the National Cholesterol Education Program (NCEP) expert panel on detection, evaluation, and treatment of high blood cholesterol in adults (Adult Treatment Panel III) (2001). Expert panel on detection, evaluation, and treatment of high blood cholesterol in adults. *JAMA*. 2001; 285: 2486–97.
2. Grundy SM, Cleeman JI, Bairey CN et al. Implications of recent clinical trials for the national cholesterol education program adult treatment panel III guidelines – 2004 update. *Circulation*. 2004; 110: 227–39.
3. Prevention of cardiovascular disease: An evidence-based clinical aid. *Med J Aust*. 2004; 181: F1–1.
4. Genest J, Frohlich J, Fodor G, McPherson R. Recommendations for the management of dyslipidemia and the prevention of cardiovascular disease: 2003 update. *CMAJ*. 2003; 169: 921–4.
5. Graham I, Atar AE, Borch-Johsen K et al. European guidelines on cardiovascular disease prevention in clinical practice. *Eur J Cardiovasc Prev Rehabil*. 2007; 14(Suppl 2): S1–113.
6. The assessment and management of cardiovascular risk. Available at http://www.nzgg.org.nz/index.cfm?fuseaction=fuseaction_10& fusesubaction=docs&documentid=22 (Accessed October 2007).
7. International Atherosclerosis Society (IAS) (2003). Harmonized guidelines on prevention of atherosclerotic cardiovascular diseases. Available at http://www.athero.org/ (Accessed October 2007).
8. Prise en charge thérapeutique du patient dyslipidémique, French Health Products Safety Agency (2005). Available at http://afssaps. sante.fr/pdf/5/rbp/dysreco.pdf (Accessed October 2007).
9. Spanish local guidelines. Available at http://www.papps.org/publicaciones/g4.htm http://www.papps.org/publicaciones/g3.html (Accessed October 2007).
10. Smith SC Jr, Jackson R, Pearson TA, Fuster V, Yusuf S, Faergeman O et al. Principles for national and regional guidelines on cardiovascular disease prevention: A scientific statement from the World Heart and Stroke Forum. *Circulation*. 2004; 109: 3112–21.
11. Yudkin P, Hey K, Roberts S et al. Abstinence from smoking eight years after participation in randomised controlled trial of nicotine patch. *BMJ*. 2003; 327: 28–9.
12. Alberti KG, Zimmet P, Shaw J. IDF epidemiology task force consensus group. The metabolic syndrome – a new worldwide definition. *Lancet*. 2005; 366: 1059–62.
13. US NHLBI website: http://nhlbisupport.com/bmi/bmicalc.htm (Accessed October 2007).
14. American Heart Association website: http://www.americanheart. org/presenter.jhtml?identifier=851 (Accessed October 2007).
15. Joint British Societies guidelines on prevention of cardiovascular disease in clinical practice. *Heart*. 2005; 91(Suppl V): v1–52.
16. Angus J, Evans S, Lapum J et al. "Sneaky disease": the body and health knowledge for people at risk for coronary heart disease in Ontario. Canada. *Soc Sci Med*. 2005; 60: 2117–28.

6

Type 2 diabetes and metabolic syndrome patients: management recommendations for reducing cardiovascular risk

F.D.R. Hobbs[1], E. McGregor[2] and J. Betteridge[3]

[1]University of Birmingham, UK
[2]The Future Forum Secretariat, London, UK
[3]University College London, London, UK

Introduction

Diabetes mellitus, in particular Type 2 diabetes but also Type 1 after the age of 40, confers substantial cardiovascular risk. In people with diabetes, at least in those who have had disease for a few years, and no history of coronary heart disease, the risk of myocardial infarction is similar to that in non-diabetic patients with manifest cardiovascular disease. However, this can depend on the current age of the patient, the presence or absence of the metabolic syndrome (Met Syn) or other cardiovascular risk factors, and the duration of Type 1 or 2 diabetes. Furthermore, both short- and long-term survival are substantially worse for diabetic patients who experience a myocardial infarction or stroke than for non-diabetic individuals. Intensive management of cardiovascular risk factors is therefore widely recommended for individuals with diabetes.

One of the metabolic defects that characterises Type 2 diabetes, insulin resistance, is also a core factor in the Met Syn (see Box 6.1 for definition of Met Syn).[1-5] In this complex disorder, hyperglycaemia and insulin resistance may exist in association with an array of lipid and non-lipid cardiovascular risk factors (Box 6.1). In a recent Scandinavian study, the Met Syn increased both the risk of cardiovascular events by three-fold and cardiovascular-related death by five- to six-fold.[6]

This article discusses the management of patients with Type 2 diabetes or Met Syn based on recommendations from the national and regional guidelines shown in Box 6.2.[7-12] Guidelines on reducing cardiovascular risk factors in diabetes patients can also be found in the diabetes guidelines summarised in Box 6.3.[13-18]

Cardiovascular Risk Management, Edited by R Hobbs and B Arroll
© 2009 Blackwell Publishing, ISBN: 9781405155755

Box 6.1 Definition of the Met Syn

Met Syn is diagnosed when ≥ 3 of the following features are present in an individual:

- Increased waist circumference ≥ 102 cm in American men, ≥ 88 cm in American women (see Figure 6.3) – this allows for rapid identification of individuals who are likely candidates for the Met Syn
- Triglycerides ≥ 1.7 mmol/L
- HDL-C <1.03 mmol/L in men, <1.3 mmol/L in women
- Blood pressure ≥ 130/85 mmHg
- Glucose ≥ 5.6 mmol/L (100 mg/dL) or known diabetic

 Source: Adapted from the Third Report of the National Cholesterol Education Program (2001), the International Atherosclerosis Society Harmonized guidelines (2003) (see Box 6.2) and the IDF definition of the Met Syn (Ref. 1).

Modifications and clarifications to the 2001 NCEP ATP III definition of the Met Syn include:

- Adjustments of waist circumference to lower thresholds (e.g. in certain ethnic groups) (see Figure 6.3).
- Reducing the threshold for counting elevated fasting glucose from ≥110 to 100 mg/dL in accordance with the American Diabetes Association's (ADA's) revised definition of impaired fasting glucose (IFG).

For revised definitions and recent critiques on the definition of the Met Syn (see: Refs 4 and 5).

Individual risk assessment for patients with diabetes or the Met Syn

The majority of the guidelines regard diabetes as a high-risk cardiovascular condition. However, there are differences in the way that diabetes is incorporated into standard risk algorithms.

Box 6.2 Regional and national guidelines for prevention of cardiovascular disease

Australia

Practical Implementation Taskforce for the Prevention of Cardiovascular Disease (2004)
Prevention of cardiovascular disease: An evidence-based clinical aid. *Med J Aust.* 2004; 181: F1–14.
http://www.mja.com.au/public/issues/181_06_200904/ful10382_fm.html

Canada

Working Group on Hypercholesterolemia and Other Dyslipidemias (2003)
Genest J, Frohlich J, Fodor G, McPherson R. Recommendations for the management of dyslipidemia and the prevention of cardiovascular disease: 2003 update. *CMAJ.* 2003; 169: 921–4.
http://www.cmaj.ca/cgi/content/full/169/9/921/DC1

Europe

Fourth Joint European Task Force (2007)
Executive Summary: Graham I, Atar AE, Borch-Johsen K et al. European guidelines on cardiovascular disease prevention in clinical practice. *Eur Heart J.* 2007; 28: 2375–414.
Full text: Graham I, Atar AE, Borch-Johsen K et al. European guidelines on cardiovascular disease prevention in clinical practice. *Eur J Cardiovasc Prev Rehabil.* 2007; 14(Suppl 2): S1–113.
http://www.escardio.org/knowledge/guidelines/CVD_Prevention_in_Clinical_Practice.htm

New Zealand

The New Zealand Guidelines Group (2003)
The assessment and management of cardiovascular risk.
http://www.nzgg.org.nz/index.cfm?fuseaction=fuseaction_10&fusesubaction=docs&documentid=22

United Kingdom

Joint British Societies JBS 2 (2005)
Joint British Societies guidelines on prevention of cardiovascular disease in clinical practice. *Heart.* 2005; 91(Suppl V): v1–52.
http://heart.bmj.com/cgi/reprint/91/suppl_5/v1

United States

National Cholesterol Education Program (2001, 2004)
Third report of the National Cholesterol Education Program (NCEP) expert panel on detection, evaluation, and treatment of high blood cholesterol in adults (Adult Treatment Panel III) (2001). Expert Panel on Detection, Evaluation, and Treatment of High Blood Cholesterol in Adults. *JAMA.* 2001; 285: 2486–97.
Grundy SM, Cleeman JI, Bairey CN et al. Implications of Recent Clinical Trials for the National Cholesterol Education Program Adult Treatment Panel III Guidelines – 2004 update.
Circulation. 2004; 110: 227–39.
http://www.nhlbi.nih.gov/guidelines/cholesterol/index.htm

International

International Atherosclerosis Society (IAS) (2003)
Harmonized guidelines on prevention of atherosclerotic cardiovascular diseases
http://www.athero.org/

For example, the NCEP ATP III guidelines view diabetes as a 'coronary heart disease-risk equivalent' and therefore eligible for secondary preventative strategies.[2,12] With few exceptions NCEP guidelines regard diabetic patients as having a 10-year coronary event risk $\geq$20%. Whilst acknowledging that the 10-year risk of some diabetic patients is <20%, the guidelines conclude that these recommendations are justified by the extremely poor prognosis of diabetic patients with manifest coronary heart disease.

This approach has not been universally adopted. As discussed by the International Atherosclerosis Society (IAS) guidelines, the absolute cardiovascular risk associated with diabetes depends on the patient's age, the type of diabetes, the duration of the diabetes and the population baseline cardiovascular risk.[3] In the United States, the 10-year coronary heart disease risk approaches or exceeds 20% in the majority of diabetic patients, and this justifies the assumption of high-risk status. However, for populations in which many diabetic patients do not have a high 10-year risk, it may be more appropriate to regard diabetic status simply as one factor among many that contribute to risk. Specifically for patients with Type 2 diabetes, the United Kingdom Prospective Diabetes Study risk calculator allows estimation of individual cardiovascular risk, weighted by glycaemic status (Box 6.4).[19–22]

The intensity of risk factor management that is appropriate for an individual diabetic patient is, to some extent, a matter of clinical judgement. The major factors that affect total cardiovascular risk in diabetic patients (Figure 6.1) should be used to determine the management strategy for each patient.

Clinical judgement is also required to determine the appropriate treatment intensity for individuals with the Met Syn, since the degree of risk associated with this condition has not been firmly established. Factors that indicate increased risk include extreme levels of Met Syn risk determinants (e.g. severe

Box 6.3 Regional and national guidelines for management of diabetes

Australia 	**National Health and Medical Research Council (2001, 2005)** National Evidence-Based Guidelines for the Management of Type 2 Diabetes Mellitus *http://www.nhmrc.gov.au/publications/synopses/di7todi13syn.htm*
Canada 	**Canadian Diabetes Association (2003)** 2003 Clinical Practice Guidelines for the Prevention and Management of Diabetes in Canada. *Can J Diabetes.* 2003; 27(Suppl 2). *http://www.diabetes.ca/cpg2003/download.aspx*
Europe 	**The Task Force on Diabetes and Cardiovascular Diseases of the European Society of Cardiology (ESC) and of the European Association for the Study of Diabetes (EASD) (2007)** Rydén L, Standl E, Bartnik M et al. Guidelines on diabetes, pre-diabetes, and cardiovascular diseases: Executive summary. *Eur Heart J.* 2007; 28: 88–136. *http://www.ncbi.nlm.nih.gov/sites/entrez?cmd=retrieve&db=pubmed&list_uids=17220161&dopt=AbstractPlus* *http://www.escardio.org/knowledge/guidelines/Diabetes_Guidelines.htm?escid=234099*
New Zealand 	**The New Zealand Guidelines Group (2003)** Evidence-based best practice guideline: Management of type 2 diabetes *http://www.nzgg.org.nz/guidelines/0036/Diabetes_full_text.pdf*
United States 	**American Diabetes Association (2006)** 2006 Clinical Practice Recommendations. Standards of Medical Care in Diabetes – 2006 *Diabetes Care.* 2006; 29(Suppl 1): S4–42. *http://care.diabetesjournals.org/content/vol29/suppl_1/*
International 	**International Diabetes Federation Clinical Guidelines Task Force (2005)** Global Guideline for Type 2 Diabetes Brussels: International Diabetes Federation, 2005 *http://www.idf.org/webdata/docs/IDF%20GGT2D.pdf*

Box 6.4. Risk calculators available online

Framingham

- Adapted by NCEP ATP III
- Risk calculator: http://hin.nhlbi.nih.gov/atpiii/calculator.asp?usertype=prof (online version)
- Risk calculator: http://hin.nhlbi.nih.gov/atpiii/riskcalc.htm (downloadable version)
- Risk calculator spreadsheet: *http://www.nhlbi.nih.gov/guidelines/cholesterol/risk_tbl.htm*
- Adapted by New Zealand Guidelines Group
  - Risk tables: http://www.nzgg.org.nz/guidelines/0035/CVD_Risk_Chart.pdf

SCORE

- SCORE risk charts: http://www.escardio.org/initiatives/prevention/SCORE+Risk+Charts.htm
- Heartscore®: http://www.escardio.org/knowledge/decision_tools/heartscore/Program+Download.htm

PROCAM

- Risk calculator: http://chdrisk.uni-muenster.de/calculator.php?iSprache=1&iVersion=1&iSiVersion=0
- Risk score: http://www.chd-taskforce.com/calculator.php?iSprache=1&iVersion=1&iSiVersion=0
- PROCAM Neuronal Network Analysis: http://chdrisk.uni-muenster.de/n_network.php?iSprache=1&iVersion=1&iSiVersion=0

UKPDS

UKPDS Risk Engine: http://www.dtu.ox.ac.uk/index.html?maindoc=/ukpds/

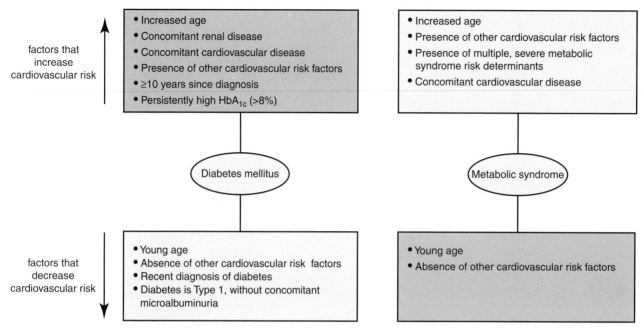

Figure 6.1 Factors that modify cardiovascular risk in patients with diabetes or the metabolic syndrome.

Risk factor		
Gender	Male	Male
Age (years)	55	65
LDL-C (mmol/L)	4.1	3.1
HDL-C (mmol/L)	1.3	1.3
Triglycerides (mmol/L)	2.3	1.6
Systolic BP (mmHg)	140	120
Family history of CVD	No	No
Diabetes mellitus	Yes	Yes
Cigarette smoker	No Yes	No Yes
10-year risk of MI or CHD death	**12% 21%**	**14% 25%**

CHD, coronary heart disease; CVD, cardiovascular disease; HDL-C, high-density lipoprotein cholesterol; LDL-C, low-density lipoprotein cholesterol; MI, myocardial infarction.

Figure 6.2 Effect of smoking on cardiovascular risk in diabetic patients. These 10-year risks were calculated using the PROCAM risk calculator which can be found at: http://chdrisk.uni-muenster.de/calculator.php?iSprache=1&iVersion=1&iSiVersion=0

obesity, very low high-density lipoprotein-cholesterol (HDL-C) levels) or additional cardiovascular risk factors (Figure 6.2). Few of the risk factors that contribute to a diagnosis of Met Syn are incorporated into the commonly used risk algorithms, although it

is increasingly accepted that they may contribute to cardiovascular risk. Many guidelines suggest that risk should first be assessed using standard algorithms but that, if a diagnosis of Met Syn is made, the patient's 10-year risk should be adjusted upwards.

Treatment goals in patients with type 2 diabetes or Met Syn

The recommended goals for patients with diabetes mellitus or Met Syn (Tables 6.1–6.4) are discussed below. These are based on the national and regional guidelines shown in Box 6.2.

In general, recommendations for patients with diabetes are similar to those for other high-risk individuals. The importance of achieving target lipid, blood pressure and glucose levels in this population means that pharmacological management is frequently required. In contrast, management of the Met Syn is based on lifestyle changes that aim to reduce the underlying causes, which include obesity and physical inactivity.[23] For these patients, it is usually recommended that pharmacological agents are introduced only if lifestyle changes fail to effect the desired improvements.

Lipid level improvements

The lipid profile of individuals with diabetes or the Met Syn is frequently characterised by elevated levels of triglycerides, small dense low-density lipoprotein (sdLDL) particles and low levels of HDL-C. However, low-density lipoprotein-cholesterol (LDL-C) generally remains the primary lipid-related target of

Table 6.1 Management of risk factors in individuals with diabetes – goals/treatments included in guideline recommendations

Goal or treatment	Guideline (see Box 6.2 for full reference)					
	Australia	Canada	Europe	New Zealand	United States	International
Smoking cessation	✓	–	✓	✓	–	✓
Lifestyle change[a]	✓	✓	✓	✓	✓[b]	✓
Dyslipidaemia	✓	✓	✓	✓	✓	✓
Hypertension	✓	–	✓	✓	–	✓
Hyperglycaemia	–	–	✓	✓	–	✓

[a]Non-atherogenic diet, achievement of optimal bodyweight, increased physical activity.
[b]If LDL-C $\geq$ 2.6 mmol/L or, regardless of LDL-C, if the individual has lifestyle-related risk factors (e.g. obesity, physical inactivity, elevated triglycerides, low HDL-C).
For patients with a history of coronary heart disease, the use of beta-blockers and angiotensin converting enzyme inhibitors is recommended by most guidelines.

Table 6.2 Lipid level goals in individuals with diabetes

Guideline	Lipid level goals	
	Threshold for initiating treatment[a]	Goal[b]
Australia	TC: 3.5 mmol/L	TC: <3.5 mmol/L
Canada	Treatment recommended in all patients	LDL-C: <2.5 mmol/L TC:HDL-C ratio: <4.0
Europe	TC: 5.0 mmol/L LDL-C: 3.0 mmol/L	TC: <4.5 mmol/L LDL-C: <2.5 mmol/L
New Zealand		TC: <4.0 mmol/L LDL-C: <2.5 mmol/L HDL-C: >1.0 mmol/L TC:HDL-C ratio: <4.5 TG: <1.7 mmol/L
United Kingdom	10-year CV risk $\geq$ 20%	LDL-C: <2.0 mmol/L TC: <4.0 mmol/L Non-HDL: <3.0 mmol/L
United States	LDL-C: 1.8–3.4[d] mmol/L	↓ by 30–40% and to <1.8, 2.6 or 3.4[d] Non-HDL-C: <2.6–4.1[c,d]
International	LDL-C: 2.6 mmol/L	LDL-C: <2.5 mmol/L Non-HDL-C: <2.6–4.1[c]

[a]Threshold for initiating lipid-modifying drugs.
[b]Even if no HDL-C and triglyceride targets are stated, attempts should be made to improve levels of these risk factors in appropriate patients.
[c]Non-HDL-C should be identified as a target only if triglycerides $\geq$2.3 mmol/L.
[d]Goal/cutpoint depends on disease status/level of risk.

Table 6.3 Lipid goals in individuals with Met Syn[a]

Guideline		Lipid level goals	
		Threshold for initiating treatment[a]	Goal[b]
🏴	**Australia**	TC: 8.0 mmol/L TC:HDL-C ratio: 8.0 mmol/L	
🍁	**Canada**		LDL-C: <3.5 or 4.5 mmol/L[e] TC:HDL-C ratio: <5.0 or 6.0[e] mmol/L
🏴	**Europe**		TC: <5.0 mmol/L LDL-C: <3.0 mmol/L
🏴	**New Zealand**	TC: 8.0 mmol/L[e] TC:HDL-C ratio: 8.0 mmol/L[e]	TC is DI LDL-C is DI HDL-C: >1.0 mmol/L TC:HDL-C ratio is DI TG is DI
🏴	**United States**	LDL-C: 3.4 or 4.1[e] mmol/L	Non-HDL-C is DI LDL-C: <3.4 mmol/L Non-HDL-C: <4.1 mmol/L[d]
🌐	**International**	LDL-C: 3.4 or 4.1[e] mmol/L	LDL-C: <3.4 mmol/L Non-HDL-C: <4.1 mmol/L[d]

[a] These goals assume a 10-year coronary event risk <20%.
[b] Threshold for initiating lipid-modifying drugs.
[c] Even if no HDL-C and triglyceride targets are stated, attempts should be made to improve levels of these risk factors in appropriate patients.
[d] Non-HDL-C should be identified as a target only if triglycerides ≥ 2.3 mmol/L.
[e] Goal/cutpoint depends on disease status/level of risk.
DI, determined individually (goals should be determined individually for each patient, according to level of risk).

Table 6.4 Blood pressure goals in individuals with diabetes or Met Syn

Guideline		Blood pressure goal (mmHg)	
		Diabetes mellitus	Metabolic syndrome
🏴	**Australia**	<130/85	<150/95
🍁	**Canada**	–	–
🏴	**Europe**	<130/80	<140/90
🏴	**New Zealand**	<130/80[a]	<140/85
🏴	**United States**	–	–
🌐	**International**	<130/85	<140/90

[a] Lower target (e.g. <120/75 mm Hg) may be recommended in patients with concomitant renal disease.

drug therapy as reducing LDL-C holds vast possibilities in preventing cardiovascular disease and thereby improving quality of life and life expectancy. Nevertheless, the lipid-lowering strategy should include efforts to lower triglyceride and increase HDL-C levels, as has been shown to be beneficial in patients treated with a statin.[6]

Lipid targets for diabetic patients are almost identical to those recommended for other high-risk patients (Table 6.2). Patients with diabetes and with a history of cardiovascular disease are at particularly high risk, and the NCEP ATP III guidelines recommend an LDL-C goal of <1.8 mmol/L for this group.[2] This is lower than the goal recommended for most other high-risk patients (<2.6 mmol/L). The Joint British Guideline 2 recommendations, which are based on recent trial results, are in line with other recent recommendations, and advocate an LDL-C target of <2 mmol/L.[11]

Few guidelines state specific lipid goals for individuals with the Met Syn. Since it is generally agreed that the Met Syn is not a 'high-risk' condition *per se*, lipid goals for individuals at 'moderate' risk (i.e. 10-year coronary event risk <20%) are appropriate for most patients with Met Syn (Table 6.3). However, if

Table 6.5 HbA$_{1c}$ goals in individuals with diabetes

Guideline		HbA$_{1c}$ (%)
	Australia	–
	Canada	–
	Europe	≤6.1
	New Zealand	≤7
	United States	–
	International	≤7

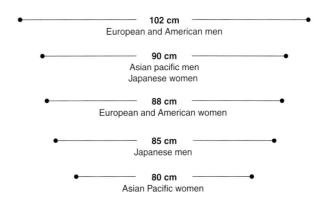

Figure 6.3 Gender- and ethnicity-based cutoffs for increased waist circumference. To define the level at which waist circumference is measured locate the hip bone (ileac crest) and lower rib and place a measuring tape at the mid-point between the two, around the abdomen, in a horizontal plane and at the diameter of maximum dimension. The plane of the tape is parallel to the floor and the tape is snug, but does not compress the skin. The measurement is made at a normal minimal respiration.

present in combination with other risk factors (e.g. hypercholesterolaemia, cigarette smoking), the Met Syn may increase 10-year risk from moderate to high (10-year risk ≥20%).

Reduction of high blood pressure

The blood pressure targets recommended for diabetic patients are generally lower than for any other patient group (Table 6.4). For example, the European guidelines recommend targets of <130/80 mmHg in diabetic patients and <140/90 mmHg in all other high-risk individuals.[9] This difference reflects the high priority given to minimising the risk of macrovascular and microvascular disease in these individuals, and the poor prognosis of diabetic patients who experience a cardiovascular event. Furthermore there are empirical data from the Hypertension Optimal Treatment (HOT) trial that show that significantly better outcomes are achieved in diabetic patients reaching the lower blood pressure targets than the levels acceptable for most hypertensive patients.[24]

Most of the guidelines do not state specific blood pressure targets for individuals with the Met Syn. The target levels shown in Table 6.5 reflect each guideline's assessment of the risk posed by the Met Syn and the blood pressure goals recommended for that risk group. The recommended target is generally <140/90 mmHg.

Bodyweight reduction

Reduction of bodyweight to within the normal range (body mass index (BMI) <25 kg/m^2) is recommended for individuals at all levels of risk. Intensity of risk factor management should always be linked to total risk, and weight reduction is therefore particularly important in overweight diabetic patients.

Increased BMI undoubtedly contributes to increased cardiovascular risk. However, it is becoming increasingly apparent that risk is affected by body fat distribution and that abdominal fat is

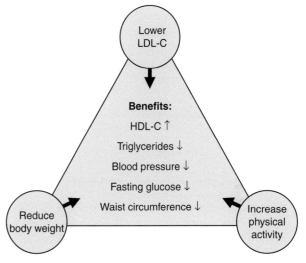

HDL-C, high-density lipoprotein cholesterol;
LDL-C, low-density lipoprotein cholesterol.

Figure 6.4 Management of the metabolic syndrome
HDL-C, high-density lipoprotein cholesterol; LDL-C, low-density lipoprotein cholesterol

particularly detrimental. Since abdominal obesity is one of the diagnostic criteria of the Met Syn (Figure 6.3), these patients are particular targets for weight loss programmes.

Increased physical activity can help patients to achieve significant weight loss. It also forms an integral part of therapy for the Met Syn, since the factors that contribute to a diagnosis of Met Syn all respond to a combination of weight reduction and increased physical activity. In combination with LDL-C reduction, these strategies form the basis of management of Met Syn (Figure 6.4).

Table 6.6 Dietary carbohydrate: recommendations for individuals with diabetes or the Met Syn

Recommendation	Diabetes mellitus	Metabolic syndrome
Include ≥ 1 serving of a low GI/high-fibre food at each meal	✓	✓
Most servings should consist of moderate–low GI and high-fibre foods	✓	✓
Distribute carbohydrate intake evenly throughout the day	✓	✓
Avoid large volumes of carbohydrate-rich food	✓	✓
Consume ≥ 40 g dietary fibre per day	✓	✓
Consume ≤ 15 g added sugar per day	✓	–

 Source: Adapted from the guidelines of the New Zealand Guidelines Group, National Heart Foundation and Stroke Foundation (2003) (see Box 6.2).

Table 6.7 Recommendations for the use of anti-thrombotic therapy

Guideline		Low-dose aspirin recommended	
		Diabetes mellitus	Metabolic syndrome
	Australia	✓	Only if 10-year risk ≥ 20%
	Canada	–	–
	Europe	✓	Only if patient has history of CHD
	New Zealand	Only if 10-year risk ≥ 20%	Only if 10-year risk ≥ 20%
	United States	–	Only if patient has history of CHD
	International	✓	✓

CHD, coronary heart disease.
The New Zealand guidelines use a 5-year risk of 15% for cardiovascular disease
risk, which approximates a 10-year 20% risk of coronary heart disease.

Dietary improvements

In general, the guidelines do not recommend specific dietary strategies for patients with diabetes or the Met Syn. Instead, guidelines recommend that all patients at increased cardiovascular risk follow a cardioprotective diet (see article in series, High-risk patients: management recommendations). The New Zealand guidelines do, however, make specific dietary recommendations for control of hyperglycaemia (see below) and the NCEP ATP III 2001 guidelines (Box 6.2) discuss dietary recommendations.[2,10]

Reduce hyperglycaemia/insulin resistance

In patients with diabetes, there is a strong link between the incidence of microvascular disease and blood glucose control. Although less well established, there is also evidence of a link with macrovascular disease. As a result, it is generally recommended that hyperglycaemia should be controlled to maintain HbA_{1c} ≤6 or 7% (Table 6.5).

There are no specific targets for control of insulin resistance or hyperglycaemia in individuals with the Met Syn. However, improvements in lifestyle (e.g. improved diet, increased physical activity) can normalise glucose tolerance and prevent or delay the onset of diabetes. As emphasised by the New Zealand guidelines, hyperglycaemia, hyperinsulinaemia, insulin resistance and HbA_{1c} levels can be substantially improved using dietary control alone (Table 6.6).[10]

Conclusions

With few exceptions, patients with diabetes mellitus should receive intensive management of cardiovascular risk factors.

Determining the appropriate treatment intensity for individuals with the Met Syn is more difficult, since this condition, and the underlying risk factors that cause it, have not been incorporated into standard risk algorithms. Clinical judgment is thus of paramount importance in these cases.

References

1. Alberti KG, Zimmet P, Shaw J. IDF Epidemiology task force consensus group. The metabolic syndrome – a new worldwide definition. *Lancet*. 2005; 366: 1059–62.
2. Expert Panel on Detection, Evaluation, and Treatment of High Blood Cholesterol in Adults. Third report of the National Cholesterol Education Program (NCEP) expert panel on detection, evaluation, and treatment of high blood cholesterol in adults (Adult Treatment Panel III) (2001). *JAMA*. 2001; 285: 2486–97.
3. International Atherosclerosis Society (IAS) (2003). Harmonized guidelines on prevention of atherosclerotic cardiovascular diseases. Available at http://www.athero.org/ (Accessed October 2007).
4. Grundy SM, Cleeman JI, Daniels SR, Donato KA, Eckel RH, Franklin BA, Gordon DJ, Krauss RM, Savage PJ, Smith SC Jr, Spertus JA, Costa F. Executive Summary. Diagnosis and management of the metabolic syndrome: An American Heart Association/ National Heart, Lung, and Blood Institute scientific statement. *Curr Opin Cardiol*. 2006; 21: 1–6.
5. Kahn R, Buse J, Ferrannini E, Stern M. American Diabetes Association; European Association for the Study of Diabetes. The metabolic syndrome: Time for a critical appraisal: Joint statement from the American Diabetes Association and the European Association for the Study of Diabetes. *Diabetes Care*. 2005; 28: 2289–304.
6. Pyörälä K, Ballantyne CM, Gumbiner B, Lee MW, Shah A, Davies MJ et al. Reduction of cardiovascular events by simvastatin in nondiabetic coronary heart disease patients with and without the metabolic syndrome: Subgroup analyses of the Scandinavian Simvastatin Survival Study (4S). *Diabetes Care*. 2004; 27: 1735–40.
7. Fulcher GR, Amarena JV, Conner GW, Gilbert RE, Hankey GJ. Practical Implementation Taskforce for the Prevention of Cardiovascular Disease. Prevention of cardiovascular disease: An evidence-based clinical aid. *Med J Aust*. 2004; 20; 181(Suppl 6): F4–14.
8. Genest J, Frohlich J, Fodor G, McPherson R. Recommendations for the management of dyslipidemia and the prevention of cardiovascular disease: 2003 update. *CMAJ*. 2003; 169: 921–4.
9. Graham I, Atar AE, Borch-Johsen K et al. European guidelines on cardiovascular disease prevention in clinical practice. *Eur J Cardiovasc Prev Rehabil*. 2007; 14(Suppl 2): S1–113.
10. New Zealand Guidelines Group. The assessment and management of cardiovascular risk (2003). Available at http://www.nzgg.org.nz/ index.cfm?fuseaction=fuseaction_10&fusesubaction=docs&docu mentid=22 (Accessed October 2007).
11. Joint British Societies guidelines on prevention of cardiovascular disease in clinical practice. *Heart*. 2005; 91(Suppl V): v1–52.
12. Grundy SM, Cleeman JI, Bairey CN, et al. Implications of recent clinical trials for the national cholesterol education program adult treatment panel III guidelines – 2004 update. *Circulation*. 2004; 110: 227–39.
13. Australian Centre for Diabetes Strategies for the Diabetes Australia Guideline Development Consortium. National evidence-based guidelines for the management of type 2 diabetes mellitus (2005). Available at *http://www.nhmrc.gov.au/publications/synopses/ di7todi13syn.htm* (Accessed October 2007).
14. Canadian Diabetes Association Clinical Practice Guidelines Expert Committee. Canadian Diabetes Association 2003 Clinical Practice Guidelines for the Prevention and Management of Diabetes in Canada. *Can J Diabetes*. 2003; 27(Suppl 2): S1–152.
15. Rydén L, Standl E, Bartnik M et al. Guidelines on diabetes, pre-diabetes, and cardiovascular diseases: Executive summary. *Eur Heart J*. 2007; 28: 88–136.
16. New Zealand Guidelines Group (2003). Evidence-based best practice guideline: Management of type 2 diabetes. Available at *http:// www.nzgg.org.nz/guidelines/0036/Diabetes_full_text.pdf* (Accessed October 2007).
17. American Diabetes Association (2006). Clinical practice recommendations. Standards of medical care in diabetes – 2006. *Diabetes Care*. 2006; 29(Suppl 1): S4–42.
18. International Diabetes Federation. Global guideline for type 2 diabetes (2005). Available at *http://www.idf.org/webdata/docs/ IDF%20GGT2D.pdf* (Accessed October 2007).
19. United Kingdom prospective diabetes study risk calculator. Available at http://www.dtu.ox.ac.uk (Accessed October 2007).
20. Framingham heart study. Available at http://www.framinghamheart-study.org/about/index.html (Accessed October 2007).
21. Conroy RM, Pyorala K, Fitzgerald AP, Sans S, Menotti A, De Backer G et al. Estimation of ten-year risk of fatal cardiovascular disease in Europe: The SCORE project. *Eur Heart J*. 2003; 24(11): 987–1003.
22. Cullen P, Schulte H, Assmann G. The Münster Heart Study (PROCAM). Total mortality in middle-aged men is increased at low total and LDL cholesterol concentrations in smokers but not in non-smokers. *Circulation*. 1997; 96: 2128–36.
23. Tuomilehto J, Lindstrom J, Eriksson JG, Valle TT, Hamalainen H, Ilanne-Parikka P et al. Prevention of type 2 diabetes mellitus by changes in lifestyle among subjects with impaired glucose tolerance. *N Engl J Med*. 2001; 344: 1343–50.
24. Hansson L, Zanchetti A, Carruthers SG, Dahlof B, Elmfeldt D, Julius S, Menard J, Rahn KH, Wedel H, Westerling S. Effects of intensive blood-pressure lowering and low-dose aspirin in patients with hypertension: Principal results of the Hypertension Optimal Treatment (HOT) randomised trial. HOT study group. *Lancet*. 1998; 351: 1755–62.

7 Lifestyle changes to reduce cardiovascular risk

J. Mendive[1], E. McGregor[2] and F. Sacks[3]

[1] Catalan Health Institute, Barcelona, Spain
[2] The Future Forum Secretariat, London, UK
[3] Harvard School of Public Health; Harvard Medical School; Boston, USA

Introduction

Epidemiological research has clearly established that many risk factors contribute to cardiovascular disease (CVD). Some of them are modifiable and treatment decisions are based on the level of risk determined by risk assessment (see article on Screening & identifying at-risk patients).

Positive lifestyle changes are crucial to the prevention and management of CVD, and can result in substantial risk reduction (Box 7.1). These changes can include smoking cessation interventions, a cardioprotective dietary pattern and physical activity. However, lifestyle changes are challenging for both the healthcare professional and the patient, and behavioural counselling and regular follow-ups are often required to overcome barriers, encourage adherence and assist in the achievement of long-term lifestyle goals.

This article aims to provide practitioners with a concise guide to the role and impact of lifestyle changes based on recommendations from six of the most up-to-date clinical practice guidelines for prevention of CVD (Box 7.2).[1–6]

Lifestyle treatment goals

Summarised below are the recommended lifestyle treatment goals to reduce CVD risk factors. Lifestyle change is appropriate

---

Box 7.1 Lifestyle changes that reduce cardiovascular risk

- Smoking cessation
- Achievement of healthy bodyweight (BMI, 25 kg/m2)
- Cardioprotective diet
- Increased physical activity

BMI: body mass index

---

for all risk levels, but some higher risk patients may also require pharmacological therapy to enable risk reduction targets to be achieved (see article on High-risk patients: management recommendations in this series).

Stop cigarette smoking

There is extensive evidence that smoking is strongly related to mortality, largely because of an increased risk of coronary heart disease (CHD) and stroke. It is one of the strongest risk factors for atherosclerotic disease, and has a dose-dependent effect on cardiovascular risk. Smoking cessation decreases this risk in patients with and without CHD, and risk reduction begins within months of quitting. Excess risk of CHD is reduced by half after 1 year's abstinence and the risk of a coronary event is reduced to the level of a non-smoker within 5 years.

Most practice guidelines recommend recording current and past smoking habits as part of a comprehensive cardiovascular risk assessment. They recommend that all patients who smoke should be strongly encouraged and helped to stop (Box 7.3). Evidence demonstrates that the more intense and longer lasting the intervention, the more likely the patient is to stay smoke-free; however, it is important to know that even an intervention lasting fewer than 3 minutes is effective. This evidence should encourage general practitioners to be more active in promoting short interventions even when they are affected by time constraints that sometimes apply in the primary care setting. Counselling and behavioural therapies can be effective, and in combination with nicotine replacement therapy, bupropion or varenicline.[7] Evidence suggests that pharmacological treatment combined with behavioural support will enable 20–25% of users to remain abstinent at 1-year post treatment. Even less intense measures, such as physicians advising their patients to quit smoking, can produce cessation rates of 5–10%. However, repeated intervention is often required as tobacco dependence is a chronic condition.

Box 7.2 Regional and national guidelines for prevention of CVD

| Australia | **Practical Implementation Taskforce for the Prevention of Cardiovascular Disease (2004)** |

Australia — **Practical Implementation Taskforce for the Prevention of Cardiovascular Disease (2004)**
Prevention of cardiovascular disease: An evidence-based clinical aid. *Med J Aust.* 2004; 181: F1–14.
http://www.mja.com.au/public/issues/181_06_200904/ful10382_fm.html

Canada — **Working Group on Hypercholesterolemia and Other Dyslipidemias (2003)**
Genest J, Frohlich J, Fodor G, McPherson R. Recommendations for the management of dyslipidemia and the prevention of cardiovascular disease: 2003 update. *CMAJ.* 2003; 169: 921–4.
http://www.cmaj.ca/cgi/content/full/ 169/9/921/DC1

Europe — **Third Joint European Task Force (2007)**
Executive Summary: Graham I, Atar AE, Borch-Johsen K et al. European guidelines on cardiovascular disease prevention in clinical practice. *Eur Heart J.* 2007; 28: 2375–414.
Full text: Graham I, Atar AE, Borch-Johsen K et al. European guidelines on cardiovascular disease prevention in clinical practice. *Eur J Cardiovasc Prev Rehabil.* 2007; 14(Suppl 2): S1–113.
http://www.escardio.org/knowledge/guidelines/CVD_Prevention_in_Clinical_Practice.htm

New Zealand — **The New Zealand Guidelines Group (2003)**
The assessment and management of cardiovascular risk
http://www.nzgg.org.nz/index.cfm?fuseaction=fuseaction_10&fusesubaction=docs&documentid=22

United States — **American Heart Association Nutrition Committee (2006)**
Diet and lifestyle recommendations revision 2006: A scientific statement from the American Heart Association Nutrition Committee.
Lichtenstein AH, Appel LJ, Brands M et al. and the American Heart Association Nutrition Committee. *Circulation.* 2006; 114: 82–96.
http://circ.ahajournals.org/cgi/content/full/114/1/82

International — **International Atherosclerosis Society (IAS) (2003)**
Harmonized guidelines on prevention of atherosclerotic cardiovascular diseases
http://www.athero.org/

Box 7.3 Clinical interventions for cigarette smoking

- Counselling and behavioural therapies
  - intensive health professional advice
  - self-help materials
  - organised group programmes
  - telephone counselling
- Pharmacotherapies
  - nicotine replacement therapy
  - bupropion or nortriptyline hydrochloride
  - varenicline
- Follow-up.

Healthy bodyweight

Changing lifestyles have resulted in a dramatic increase in the number of overweight and obese people worldwide.[8] Being overweight and/or suffering from obesity not only predispose to CHD, stroke, and numerous other conditions, they are also associated with greater all-cause mortality. People who are overweight or obese usually have a high burden of other CHD risk factors including dyslipidaemia (high low-density lipoprotein cholesterol (LDL-C), low high-density lipoprotein cholesterol

(HDL-C), and high triglycerides), Type 2 diabetes and hypertension. Obese individuals who do not yet have these risk factors are at an increased risk of developing them. Weight reduction is an important goal in overweight or obese individuals.

Bodyweight is most readily quantified as body mass index (Figure 7.1). Obesity is usually defined as a BMI of $\geqslant 25\,\text{kg/m}^2$ (Asian-Pacific region) and $\geqslant 30\,\text{kg/m}^2$ (Europe and United States) with regional differences occurring (Table 7.1). Cardiovascular risk is also influenced by the regional distribution of body fat and abdominal fat is particularly detrimental. Patients with abdominal obesity (commonly defined as a waist circumference $\geqslant 102\,\text{cm}$ in men, $\geqslant 88\,\text{cm}$ in women) should be encouraged to lose weight, regardless of BMI. These values are based on European populations and may not be appropriate for all age and ethnic groups (Table 7.2).[6]

Treatment for overweight or obese individuals should include counselling and help in achieving bodyweight reduction. The guidelines recommend that weight loss should be achieved through a combination of dietary modification and increased physical activity. Consideration of readiness to change and level of motivation should be assessed. Reviewing the patient's past attempts at weight loss and explaining how the new treatment plan will be different can encourage patients and provide hope for successful weight loss.

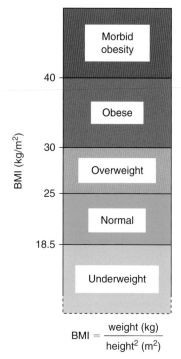

$$BMI = \frac{weight\ (kg)}{height^2\ (m^2)}$$

Figure 7.1 Body mass index (BMI). If weight reduction is necessary, energy intake should be reduced by 500–1,000 kcal/day with the initial aim of reducing bodyweight by 10% within 6 months. A BMI calculator that uses both metric and imperial measurements is available at: http://nhlbisupport.com/bmi/bmicalc.htm

Table 7.1 Classification of body weight by region

Body weight category	Europe and United States BMI	Asian-Pacific region BMI	Risk of obesity-related co-morbidities
Underweight	<18.5	<18.5	Low (risk of other clinical problems increased)
Normal	18.5–24.9	18.5–22.9	Average
Overweight (moderate risk)	25–29.9	23–24.9	Increased
Obesity	≥30	≥25	
Class I obesity	30–34.9	25–29.9	Moderate
Class II obesity	35–39.9	≥30	Severe
Class III obesity	≥40		Very severe

The goal of therapy is to achieve a healthy bodyweight (Box 7.4). Modest weight reductions are associated with significant improvements in lipid abnormalities, blood pressure levels, insulin resistance and glycaemic control. It is estimated that for every 1% decrease in body weight, triglycerides decrease by 0.01 mmol/L and HDL-C increases by 0.01 mmol/L.

Table 7.2 Population-specific recommendations for increased waist circumference

	Europe and United States	Asian-Pacific region	Japan
Men	≥102 cm (≥40 in)	≥90 cm	≥85 cm
Women	≥88 cm (≥35 in)	≥80 cm	≥90 cm

Note: International Atherosclerosis Society (IAS) (2003).

Box 7.4 Goals and strategy to manage overweight and obesity

Goals

- At a minimum, to prevent further weight gain
- Attain healthy weight
  - 5 kg weight loss or a 5–10% reduction in body weight
  - BMI <25 kg/m²
- To maintain lower body weight over the long term.

Strategy

- Ongoing counselling and group support are essential for long-term success
- Provide literature relating to BMI and health outcomes
- Discuss
  - lifestyle patterns that promote weight loss
  - portion control
  - daily/weekly physical exercise/activity
- Provide literature on product labelling, calorie content and recommended portion size
- Follow-up to examine weight/BMI and discuss barriers to adherence.

In people with elevated blood pressure, a body weight loss in the range of 5–10% is associated with an average blood pressure reduction of 3 mmHg in both systolic and diastolic pressures. However, even the loss of 3–5 pounds (approximately 1.5–2.5 kg) can make a significant difference in a patient's risk profile by improving lipids and insulin metabolism.

Improve diet

A patient's diet should be assessed to determine the level of knowledge and attitude to diet if considering the prevention of CVD. For example, the patient's current intake of saturated fat, dietary cholesterol and trans-fatty acids may help identify the potential targets for modification.

The guidelines provide recommendations on a healthy diet aimed at reducing the total calorie intake (see High-risk patients:

Table 7.3 OmniHeart trial: Estimated 10-year risk of CHD at baseline and by diet from the Framingham and PROCAM risk equations

	Baseline	Diet rich in:		
		Carbohydrate	Protein	Unsaturated fat
		CHD risk by Framingham equation (%)		
All				
Estimated 10-year CHD risk[†]	5.1	4.3	4.0	4.1
Change from baseline[‡]		−16.1	−21.0	−19.6
Change from carbohydrate-rich diet[‡]			**−5.8**	**−4.2**
Men				
Estimated 10-year CHD risk[†]	7.5	6.4	6.1	6.2
Change from baseline[‡]		−13.8	−18.7	−17.2
Change from carbohydrate-rich diet[‡]			**−5.6**	**−3.9**
Women				
Estimated 10-year CHD risk[†]	2.2	1.7	1.5	1.5
Change from baseline[‡]		−21.2	−30.0	−31.3
Change from carbohydrate-rich diet[‡]			**−11.1**	**−12.9**
		CHD risk by PROCAM equation (%)		
Men				
Estimated 10-year CHD risk[†]	6.4	5.1	4.4	4.5
Change from baseline[‡]		−20.0	−30.7	−29.4
Change from carbohydrate-rich diet[‡]			**−13.4**	**−11.8**

CHD, coronary heart disease; PROCAM, Prospective Cardiovascular Munster.

[†]Estimated percentage of individuals experiencing a CHD event over 10 years.

[‡]Estimated change in risk from baseline or carbohydrate-rich diet, expressed as a percentage.

Source: Reproduced with permission from American Medical Association. Ref. 13.

management recommendations in this series). This recommended dietary pattern includes fruits and vegetables, whole grains, fish and/or dried peas and beans or soya products, oil, spreads, nuts or seeds, low-fat milk products, and optional small servings of lean meat or skinned poultry. It avoids regular consumption of foods prepared with meat or dairy fats. This pattern of diet is known in Southern European countries as a Mediterranean diet that strongly encourages the use of vegetable oils (mainly olive oil) as a source of unsaturated fats. Several studies have shown the beneficial impact of a Mediterranean diet including olive oil and nuts on cardiovascular risk factors. These include the PREDIMED Study, the EUROLIVE Study and studies by Esposito et al.[9–11] The Dietary Approaches to Stop Hypertension (DASH) Studies showed blood pressure could be lowered by a diet rich in fruits and vegetables, with reduced saturated and total fat or with reduced sodium.[12] The OmniHeart study showed that reducing carbohydrate in an already 'healthful' diet by partially replacing it with protein or unsaturated fat can lower blood pressure, improve lipid levels and thereby reduce estimated cardiovascular risk (Table 7.3).[13]

In the Women's Health Initiative (WHI) trial in postmenopausal women, dietary intervention that reduced total fat intake and increased intake of vegetables, fruit and grains did not significantly reduce the risk of CHD, stroke or CVD.[14] However, the intervention achieved less effect on CVD risk factors than can be predicted from the dietary goals, thereby implicating low adherence. The authors suggested that a more focused diet with lifestyle interventions may be needed. The dietary approach used in the WHI trial, in which total fat was reduced rather than specifically reducing harmful fats, that is saturated and trans-fatty acids, followed from an earlier hypothesis, not confirmed by the trial itself or later studies, that any dietary fat increases breast cancer. A more contemporary approach to specifically target CVD would be to replace saturated and trans-fatty acids with mono- and polyunsaturated fats, as recommended by the American Heart Association's Nutrition Committee in 2006.[5] Fundamentally, dietary intervention should be based on dietary patterns rather than quantitative nutrient targets, since dietary patterns are practical, and easily understood. The new American Heart Association guidelines employ a dietary patterns approach and de-emphasise nutrient-based counselling.[15]

In addition, the guidelines advise on dietary constituents known to provide protection against CVD such as dietary fibre and plant stanol/sterol esters (Table 7.4).[16–18] Advice is also given on the recommended daily intake of other vitamins,

Table 7.4 Additional dietary options for cardiovascular health

Nutrient	Recommended intake (per day)	Evidence to support cardiovascular health
Viscous fibre	5–10 g	Reduces LDL-C by about 3–4%
Plant stanols/sterol	2–3 g	Reduces LDL-C by 6–15%
Folic acid	400 μg	Supplements not effective in randomised controlled trials of CV risk reduction
Antioxidants		
vitamin C	75 mg women	Evidence does not support
vitamin E	90 mg men 15 mg	benefit of supplements
Minerals		
sodium reduction	<2,400 mg (6 g	Lowers blood pressure
potassium	sodium chloride) 90 mmol	reduces CVD
Herbal, botanical and dietary supplements	Use not recommended	No clinical trial evidence to support use

Note: Practical dietary guidelines for patients that provide recommendations similar to those above are available at the American Heart Association website: http://www.americanheart.org/presenter. jhtml?identifier=851

Box 7.5 Physical activity in healthy adults

Examples of moderate physical activity

- Brisk walking (3–4 mph) for 30–40 minutes
- Swimming – laps for 20 minutes
- Bicycling, 5 miles in 30 minutes
- Volleyball for 45 minutes
- Raking leaves for 30 minutes
- Moderate lawn mowing (not motorised) for 30 minutes
- Home care: heavy cleaning
- Basketball for 15–20 minutes
- Golf – pulling a cart or carrying clubs
- Social dancing for 30 minutes

Example of incorporating physical activity into the day

- Walk more, for example
  - Park farther away in parking lots near mall or at work
  - Walk or bike if destination a short distance away
  - Walk up stairs instead of using the elevator or escalator
  - Walk after work for 30 minutes before getting in the car
  - Walk with a colleague at the start of lunch for 20 minutes
  - Get off bus or underground one stop early and walk
- Do heavy house cleaning, push a stroller, take walks with children
- Exercise at home while watching television
- Go dancing or join an exercise programme

 Source: Adapted from the Third Report of the National Cholesterol Education Program (2001).

minerals and supplements, but currently there is insufficient evidence to support their effects on cardiovascular events.

Moderate alcohol consumption is associated with lower mortality, and higher consumption with higher mortality. Therefore the guidelines recommend moderate consumption of around two drinks (20 g of alcohol) per day for men and one drink per day for women. This gender distinction takes into account differences in both weight and metabolism, and the association in women between alcohol intake and breast cancer.

The benefits of lifestyle interventions are limited by the difficulties in maintaining weight loss. Within 3–5 years of achieving targets during an intensive, individually tailored weight loss programme, 13–38% of people have regained the weight lost. It must be recognised that the 'natural' untreated outcome is continued weight gain from baseline, so intervention likely produces a net benefit.

Effective interventions combine nutrition education with behaviourally oriented counselling to help people acquire the skills, motivation and support needed to alter their daily eating patterns and food preparation attitudes. Counselling from a primary healthcare professional or qualified dietician and frequent follow-up to examine weight/BMI and help overcome barriers to adherence can assist the long-term goals of any weight management programme. Some of the guidelines recommend pharmacotherapy for obese individuals and surgery to aid weight reduction when all other measures have failed.

Increase physical activity

Over 60% of the world's population is sedentary and not sufficiently physically active to gain the health benefits of exercise. Physical inactivity further contributes to overweight/obesity, moreover, regular physical activity enhances dietary-induced weight loss and the maintenance of weight loss, favourably modifies several risk factors; including lowering LDL-C and triglyceride levels, raising HDL-C, improving insulin sensitivity and lowering blood pressure. In addition, it is associated with reduced risk of CVD morbidity and mortality.

The guidelines recommend that all patients should be encouraged and supported to increase their physical activity safely to the level associated with the lowest risk of CVD. Healthy people should be advised to increase their physical activity based on a patient's cardiac status, age and other factors. The goal of therapy is at least 30 minutes of physical activity most days of the week, although more moderate activity is also associated with health benefits. Physicians can provide specific advice regarding types of exercise and how to integrate activities into a person's lifestyle (Box 7.5).[19] In high-risk patients, the recommended level of physical exertion should be based on the

Box 7.6   Strategy to enhance the effectives of behavioural counselling

- Develop a therapeutic alliance with the patient
- Ensure that patients understand the relationship between behaviour, health and disease
- Help patients to understand the barriers to behavioural change
- Gain commitments from patients to behavioural change
- Involve patients in identifying and selecting the risk factors to change
- Use a combination of strategies including reinforcement of patients' own capacity for change
- Design a lifestyle modification plan (specific for the individual)
- Monitor progress through follow-up contact (fix appointments)
- Involve other healthcare staff wherever possible (nurses)

 Source: Adapted from Third Joint Task Force of European and other Societies on Cardiovascular Disease Prevention in Clinical Practice.

results of a comprehensive clinical evaluation; the inclusion of an exercise test in this evaluation is discretionary.

Follow-up visits to monitor physical activity level are important to ensure long-term adherence. In addition, follow-up counselling may be required to discuss barriers to physical activity.

Putting lifestyle changes into practice

Lifestyle changes are integral to the prevention and treatment of CVD, and can result in substantial risk reduction. However, these changes are challenging for both the clinician and the patient. Behavioural counselling can help people acquire the skills, motivation and support needed to alter their daily lifestyles (Box 7.6). Patient education and motivation are vital, and communication with the patient is fundamental to successful implementation and achievement of long-term lifestyle goals. Recent surveys suggest a serious gap between the need for recommendations for behavioural change and the advice provided by physicians in routine clinical practice. Techniques that encourage patient compliance will be discussed later in this series.

Treatment approaches for high-risk patients

Many risk factors can be modified by lifestyle changes, which form the basis of risk reduction for all patients. In high-risk patients, adequate improvement in risk profile is rarely achieved using non-pharmacological management alone. Depending on the individual's risk profile, lipid-modifying,

antihypertensive and antihyperglycaemic medication may also be required (see articles on High-risk patients: Management of recommendations and Type 2 diabetes in this series).

Psychosocial factors

The cardiovascular health of patients may be affected by psychosocial factors including depression and social isolation in addition to physical factors. The guidelines recognise the importance of identifying these factors during risk assessment. Physicians play an important role in ensuring such patients receive appropriate help. More research is needed to clearly identify the relationship between psychosocial factors and CVD, as well as to define the positive impact of lifestyle changes on psychosocial health.

Conclusion

Management of cardiovascular health of patients requires changes in many patterns of individual behaviour. These behaviour changes are similar for those at low and at high risk and can result in substantial risk reduction. The challenge for physicians is to encourage patients to achieve and sustain these changes.

References

1. Prevention of cardiovascular disease: An evidence-based clinical aid. *Med J Aust.* 2004; 181: F1–14.
2. Genest J, Frohlich J, Fodor G, McPherson R. Recommendations for the management of dyslipidemia and the prevention of cardiovascular disease: 2003 update. *CMAJ.* 2003; 169: 921–4.
3. Graham I, Atar AE, Borch-Johsen K et al. European guidelines on cardiovascular disease prevention in clinical practice. *Eur J Cardiovasc Prev Rehabil.* 2007; 14(Suppl 2): S1–113.
4. The assessment and management of cardiovascular risk. Available at http://www.nzgg.org.nz/index.cfm?fuseaction=fuseaction_10&fusesubaction=docs&documentid=22 (Accessed October 2007).
5. Lichtenstein AH, Appel LJ, Brands M et al. and the American Heart Association Nutrition Committee. Diet and lifestyle recommendations revision 2006: A scientific statement from the American Heart Association Nutrition Committee. *Circulation.* 2006; 114: 82–96.
6. International Atherosclerosis Society (IAS) (2003). Harmonized guidelines on prevention of atherosclerotic cardiovascular diseases. Available at http://www.athero.org/ (Accessed October 2007).
7. West R, McNeill A, Raw M. Smoking cessation guidelines for health professionals: An update. *Thorax.* 2000; 55: 987–99.
8. WHO/FAO, *Diet, Nutrition and the Prevention of Chronic Diseases: Report of a Joint WHO/ FAO Expert Consultation.* Geneva, Switzerland, WHO, 2002.
9. Estruch R, Martinez-Gonzalez MA, Corella D et al. for the PREDIMED Study Investigators. Effects of a Mediterranean – style diet on cardiovascular risk factors: a randomized trail. *Ann Int Med.* 2006; 145(1): 1–11.
10. Covas M-I, Nyyssonen K, Poulsen HE et al. for the EUROLIVE Study Group. The effect of polyphenols in olive oil on heart

disease risk factors. A randomized trial. *Ann Int Med.* 2006; 145(5): 333–41.

11. Esposito K, Marfella R, Ciotola M et al. Effect of a Mediterranean-style diet on endothelial dysfunction and markers of vascular inflammation in the metabolic syndrome: A randomized trial. *JAMA.* 2004; 292(12): 1440–6.

12. Appel LJ, Moore TJ, Obarzanek E et al. A clinical trial of the effects of dietary patterns on blood pressure. *NEJM.* 1997; 336(16): 1117–24.

13. Appel LJ, Sacks FM, Carey VJ et al. Effects of protein, monounsaturated fat, and carbohydrate intake on blood pressure and serum lipids. Results of the OmniHeart randomized trial. *JAMA.* 2005; 294(19): 2455–64.

14. Howard BV, Van Horn L, Hsia J et al. Low-fat dietary pattern and risk of cardiovascular disease: The woman's health initiative randomized controlled dietary modification trial. *JAMA.* 2006; 295(6): 665.

15. American heart association 2006 diet and lifestyle recommendations. Available at http://www.americanheart.org/presenter.jhtml?identifier=851 (Accessed October 2007).

16. Brown L, Rosner B, Willett W, Sacks F. Cholesterol lowering effects of dietary fiber: A meta analysis. *Am J Clin Nutr.* 1999; 69: 30–42.

17. Jenkins DJ, Kendall CW, Axelsen M et al. Viscous and nonviscous fibres, nonabsorbable and low glycaemic index carbohydrates, blood lipids and coronary heart disease. *Curr Opin Lipidol.* 2000; 11: 49–56.

18. Law MR. Plant sterol and stanol margarines and health. *West J Med.* 2000; 173: 43–7.

19. Third report of the National Cholesterol Education Program (NCEP) expert panel on detection, evaluation, and treatment of high blood cholesterol in adults (Adult Treatment Panel III) (2001). Expert panel on detection, evaluation, and treatment of high blood cholesterol in adults. *JAMA.* 2001; 285: 2486–97.

8

Pharmacotherapy: improving the lipid profile

F.D.R. Hobbs[1], E. Mcgregor[2] and J. Shepherd[3]
[1]University of Birmingham, UK
[2]The Future Forum Secretariat, London, UK
[3]North Glasgow University Hospital Division, Glasgow, UK

Introduction

Epidemiological and clinical research has determined that lipids substantially contribute to cardiovascular disease (CVD) and that modifying the lipid profile has a significant impact on coronary events. These findings are reflected in continuously updated CVD management guidelines, which focus on low-density lipoprotein cholesterol (LDL-C) as the primary therapeutic target. The guidelines have further defined LDL-C levels to which patients should be treated. An individual's eligibility for treatment, and their LDL-C treatment goal and intensity of therapy is determined by their absolute CVD risk (see article on Screening & identifying at-risk patients).

Lipid abnormalities can be partly modified by lifestyle changes, which is integral to reducing risk for all patients. However, as lipid goals are progressively lowered, many patients will not be able to achieve them using non-pharmacological management alone and these patients usually require treatment with lipid-modifying drugs.

This article aims to provide practitioners with a concise guide to managing lipids with pharmacotherapy based on recommendations from six of the most up-to-date clinical practice guidelines for prevention of CVD (Box 8.1).[1–7]

Lipids and CVD

Epidemiological research has demonstrated that elevated serum total cholesterol levels are associated with an increased risk of developing coronary heart disease (CHD). Because most serum cholesterol is transported through the blood stream to tissues as LDL-C, this relationship with CHD holds true with LDL-C.

More recent large-scale intervention trials have shown a highly significant and substantial relationship between reduction of cholesterol and reduction in both mortality, due to CHD, and total mortality (Figure 8.1).[8] Indeed, data indicate that for every 1% reduction in LDL-C levels, relative risk for major CHD events is reduced by approximately 1%. This equates on average to a 20% reduction in coronary events per mmol/L fall in LDL-C. Such findings are reflected in current CVD management guidelines, which focus on LDL-C as the primary therapeutic target.

While LDL-C is important, data have also emphasised the importance of other lipids in the development of CVD, including high-density lipoprotein cholesterol (HDL-C) and triglycerides. HDL-C, through mediation of reverse cholesterol transport from peripheral tissues to the liver, is also an important regulator of CHD risk. Below average HDL-C concentrations are associated with increased CHD risk. Importantly, this relationship is independent of LDL-C level. The data indicate that a 0.025 mmol/L (1 mg/dL) increase in HDL-C reduces CHD risk by 2–4%. Elevated triglyceride levels, usually in association with reduced HDL-C concentrations, are related to increased CHD risk, although the evidence and association is weaker than for LDL-C.

Improving the lipid profile

Lifestyle changes are an integral component of the management of cardiovascular risk (see section on Lifestyle changes to reduce cardiovascular risk). Most guidelines recommend using lifestyle therapy to alter the lipid profile for around 3 months in primary prevention. After this time, if the lipid goals have not been achieved, consideration may be given to initiating

Cardiovascular Risk Management, Edited by R Hobbs and B Arroll
© 2009 Blackwell Publishing, ISBN: 9781405155755

Box 8.1 Regional and national guidelines for prevention of cardiovascular disease

Australia 	**Practical Implementation Taskforce for the Prevention of Cardiovascular Disease (2004)** Prevention of cardiovascular disease: An evidence-based clinical aid. *Med J Aust.* 2004; 181: F1–14. *http://www.mja.com.au/public/issues/181_06_200904/ful10382_fm.html*
Canada 	**Working Group on Hypercholesterolemia and Other Dyslipidemias (2003)** Genest J, Frohlich J, Fodor G, McPherson R. Recommendations for the management of dyslipidemia and the prevention of cardiovascular disease: 2003 update. *CMAJ.* 2003; 169: 921–4. *http://www.cmaj.ca/cgi/content/full/169/9/921/DC1*
Europe 	**Third Joint European Task Force (2007)** Graham I, Atar AE, Borch-Johsen K et al. European guidelines on cardiovascular disease prevention in clinical practice: Executive Summary. *Eur Heart J.* 2007; 28: 2375–414. Full text: Graham I, Atar AE, Borch-Johsen K et al. European guidelines on cardiovascular disease prevention in clinical practice. *Eur J Cardiovasc Prev Rehabil.* 2007; 14(Suppl 2): S1–113. *http://www.escardio.org/knowledge/guidelines/CVD_Prevention_in_Clinical_Practice.htm*
New Zealand 	**The New Zealand Guidelines Group (2003)** The assessment and management of cardiovascular risk *http://www.nzgg.org.nz/index.cfm?fuseaction=fuseaction_10&fusesubaction=docs&documentid=22*
USA 	**National Cholesterol Education Program (2001, 2004)** Third report of the National Cholesterol Education Program (NCEP) expert panel on detection, evaluation, and treatment of high blood cholesterol in adults (Adult Treatment Panel III) (2001). Expert panel on detection, evaluation, and treatment of high blood cholesterol in adults. *JAMA.* 2001; 285: 2486–97. Grundy SM, Cleeman JI, Bairey CN et al. Implications of recent clinical trials for the National Cholesterol Education Program Adult Treatment Panel III Guidelines – 2004 update. *Circulation* 2004; 110: 227–39. *http://www.nhlbi.nih.gov/guidelines/cholesterol/index.htm*
International	**International Atherosclerosis Society (IAS) (2003)** Harmonized guidelines on prevention of atherosclerotic cardiovascular diseases *http://www.athero.org/*

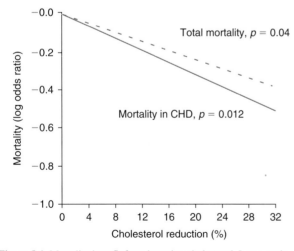

Figure 8.1 Mortality benefit from lowering cholesterol. Large-scale intervention trials have shown a clear relationship between reduction of cholesterol and reduction in both mortality, due to coronary heart disease, and total mortality. Guideline bodies have used these data to support more aggressive recommendations for treatment. *Source*: Adapted from: Ref. 8.

pharmacotherapy in conjunction with lifestyle modification (Figure 8.2).

Lifestyle changes are challenging for the patient to achieve and maintain, and a significant portion of the population will require pharmacotherapy to attain their lipid goals. In addition, those individuals at high risk, such as those who have already suffered events, or who have marked hypercholesterolaemia should commence pharmacotherapy simultaneously with lifestyle changes.

Statins and other lipid-lowering agents

Lipids can be altered by a number of drugs (Table 8.1). The lipid profile will determine the drug treatment required to lower lipid levels. The guidelines recommend HMG-CoA reductase inhibitors (statins) as the first-line treatment if the main abnormality is elevated LDL-C. Extensive clinical trial data have demonstrated that they are the most effective pharmacotherapy for lowering LDL-C and statin-mediated LDL-C reductions are associated with significant improvements in cardiovascular outcomes (Table 8.2).[9]

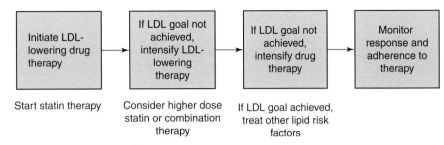

Figure 8.2 Initiation of LDL-lowering pharmacotherapy.[5]

   Source: Adapted from the Third Report of the National Cholesterol Education Program (2001); produced by the NHLBI (part of the NIH and the US Department of Health & Human Services. Available at: http://www.nhlbi.nih.gov/guidelines/cholesterol/index.htm

Table 8.1 Effects of pharmacotherapy on lipids

Drug class	LDL-C (%)	HDL-C (%)	Triglycerides (%)
Statins*	↓ 18–55	↑ 5–15	↓ 7–30
Bile acid sequestrants	↓ 15–30	↑ 3–5	No change
Nicotinic acid	↓ 5–25	↑ 15–35	↓ 20–50
Fibrates	↓ 5–20	↑ 10–20	↓ 20–50
Cholesterol absorption inhibitors	↓ 18	↑ 1	↓ 8

*Excludes rosuvastatin.

   Source: Data from the Third Report of the National Cholesterol Education Program (2001); produced by the NHLBI (part of the NIH and the US Department of Health & Human Services. Available at: http://www.nhlbi.nih.gov/guidelines/cholesterol/index.htm
Zetia prescribing information, http://www.zetia.com/zetia/shared/documents/zetia_pi.pdf

The selection of statin and starting dose will depend on the baseline LDL-C level. The guidelines recommend using a dose that can achieve a reduction in risk for major coronary events of 30–40% (Table 8.3). However, the response of an individual may vary considerably (Box 8.2). In addition, there is a tendency in current clinical practice to initiate therapy at the usual starting dose, but the dose often is not titrated upwards to achieve target goals. Persons requiring large LDL reductions will not achieve target goals with the starting dose of some statins. Furthermore, significant differences exist between statins in their efficacy at lowering LDL, although side effects are comparable and effects on other lipid variables are more predictable.[10,11] Deciding on which statin to use is guided in most countries by a balance between cost and efficacy and the importance of direct outcome data for specific agents.

If the treatment goal has been achieved at follow-up, the current dose can be maintained. If the goal has not been attained, the LDL-lowering therapy should be intensified either by increasing the statin dose or combining with another therapy.

Table 8.2 Benefit of LDL-C reduction on coronary events

Trial	Statin	n	Follow up	LDL-C reduction from baseline (%)	Reduction in major coronary event (%)
Primary prevention					
AFCAPS/TexCAPS	Lovastatin	6,605	5.2 years	−25	−37
ASCOT-LLA	Atorvastatin	10,305	3.3 years*	−35**	−37
WOSCOPS	Pravastatin	6,595	4.9 years	−26	−31
Secondary prevention					
4S	Simvastatin	4,444	5.4 years	−35	−34
CARE	Pravastatin	4,159	5 years	−32	−24
HPS	Simvastatin	20,536	5.5 years	−38	−27
LIPID	Pravastatin	9,014	6.1 years	−25**	−24
PROVE-IT	Pravastatin	4,162	2 years	−10	
	Atorvastatin			−42	−16 vs prava
TNT	Atorvastatin	10,001	4.9 years	−35	−22 vs atorva 10 mg
Ischaemia					
AVERT	Atorvastatin	341	18 months	−46	−36***
LIPS	Fluvastatin	1,677	3.9 years	−27	−20
MIRACL	Atorvastatin	3,086	16 wks	−40	−16***

* Stopped early; **vs placebo; *** AVERT & MIRACL did not show significant reductions in hard CHD endpoints; both were short-term trials and were not powered to show such a difference.

Table 8.3 Doses of statins required to attain 30–40% reduction of LDL-C levels

Statin	Dose (mg/d)	LDL reduction (%)
Fluvastatin	40–80	25–35
Lovastatin	40	31
Pravastatin	40	34
Simvastatin	20–40	35–41
Atorvastatin	10	39
Rosuvastatin	5–10	39–45

Box 8.2 Influences on LDL response to pharmacotherapy

- Diet and drug compliance
- Body weight
- Genetic cause of hypercholesterolaemia
- Gender
- Hormonal status
- Apo E phenotype
- Differences in drug absorption and metabolism.

In general, for every doubling of a statin dose, LDL levels only fall by a further 5–7%. Combination therapy however can decrease LDL-C levels by an additional 10–20%. Options include bile acid sequestrants, cholesterol absorption inhibitors and fibrates. Fibrates are primarily employed to lower triglyceride levels in patients with isolated hypertriglyceridaemia. They may be added to statin therapy where target levels have not been achieved with statin alone. Unfortunately, the findings of the FIELD Study[12] which used this combination in diabetic subjects, suggest that cardiovascular risk was not uniformly improved, particularly in individuals who had reached LDL cholesterol target with statins alone. While cardiovascular events were reduced by combination treatment, total mortality over the 5 year study did not improve. The cholesterol absorption inhibitor ezetimibe is better tolerated than bile acid sequestrants and therefore a preferred option for most patients. Ezetimibe combined with a statin can produce additional 20% reductions in LDL-C, with minor falls in triglyceride levels (approx. 6–9%) and a small increase in HDL-C (approx. 3%).[13] Again, however, use of this combination produced some disquiet in enhance.[14] Seven hundred and twenty individuals with familial hypercholesterolaemia contributed to this double-blind placebo controlled trial of a simvastatin/ezetimibe combination. This treatment did not induce any improvement in carotid intima-media thickness over a two year study period when compared to statin alone. The study was not powered to demonstrate clinical outcome benefits (ie reductions in vascular events) and until studies with that objective are reported, it may be prudent to encourage patients who do not reach LDL cholesterol targets with statin therapy alone to redouble their efforts to optimize their diet and expand their exercise program. Alternatively, nicotinic acid can also be used in combination with a statin to achieve lipid goals. However, careful slow dose-titration of nicotinic acid needs to be performed at initiation to reduce the effects of adverse side effects.

Once the LDL-C goal has been attained, attention turns to other lipid goals and risk factors, when present.

Lipid intervention goals

The guidelines recommend target LDL-C levels. The basic principle guiding treatment goals is related to risk (Table 8.4). People at the highest risk, such as those with CHD, have the lowest goal and receive the most intensive treatment. All the guidelines recommend an LDL-C goal of <2.6 mmol/L for high-risk patients.

A number of recent clinical trials, including Pravastatin or Atorvastatin Evaluation and Infection Therapy (PROVE-IT) and Treating to New Targets (TNT), have failed to identify an LDL-C threshold level below which no further cardiovascular risk reduction occurs (Figure 8.3), at least in secondary prevention.[15,16,17] Such findings suggest lower LDL-C goals than currently recommended in most of the guidelines. On this basis, the United States National Cholesterol Education Program (US-NCEP) recommended that the LDL-C goal in people at very high risk (those with prior CHD and multiple risk factors, especially diabetes) be lowered from the 2.6 to 1.8 mmol/L.[5,6]

In addition, specific patient groups, such as those with diabetes, may have intensified goals (see section on Type 2 diabetes and metabolic syndrome patients – management recommendations for reducing cardiovascular risk).

Some guidelines also highlight secondary goals of therapy, including the HDL-C/total cholesterol ratio and non-HDL-C (Table 8.5). In addition, most of the guidelines regard a triglyceride level <1.7 mmol/L as preferable, although it is not considered a specific treatment goal. Optimal HDL-C levels are rarely stated, but there is widespread agreement that cardiovascular risk is increased by HDL-C levels <1.0 mmol/L (men) and <1.3 mmol/L (women).

Monitoring

Prior to initiating drug therapy, baseline lipid measurements that will be used to follow the drug's efficacy and safety should be documented. Measurements should also include liver function tests (i.e. alanine aminotransferase or ALT, and aspartate aminotransferase or AST) and creatine kinase (CK) and an appropriate medical history should be taken (Table 8.6). All

Table 8.4 Lipid goals

Guideline	Cutpoint for initiating lipid modifying drugs	Risk level	Goal[a] (mmol/L)			
			LDL-C	TC	TC: HDL-C ratio	Non-HDL-C
Australia	TC: 3.5/5.0 mmol/L[b]	High	–	<3.5/5.0	–	–
		Intermediate	–	–	–	–
		Low	–	<6.5/7.5	–	–
Canada	Treatment recommended in all patients	High	<2.5	–	<4.0	–
		Intermediate	<3.5	–	<5.0	–
		Low	<4.5	–	<6.0	–
Europe	LDL-C: 3.0 mmol/L	High	<2.5	<4.5	used to estimate risk	–
		Intermediate	<3.0	<5.0		–
		Low	<3.0	<5.0		–
New Zealand	TC: 8.0 mmol/L TC: HDL-C: 8.0	High	<2.5[c]	<4.0[c]	<4.5[c]	–
		Intermediate	<2.5[c]	<4.0[c]	<4.0[c]	–
		Low	<2.5[c]	<4.0[c]	<4.0[c]	–
United States	LDL-C: 2.6 mmol/L (optional if LDL-C<2.6 mmol/L)	High	<1.8/2.6	–	–	<3.4[d]
		Intermediate	<3.4	–	–	<3.4[d]
		Low	<4.1	–	–	<3.4[d]
International	LDL-C: 2.6 mmol/L (optional if LDL-C<2.6 mmol/L)	High	<2.6	–	–	<3.4[d]
		Intermediate	<3.4	–	–	<3.4[d]
		Low	<4.1	–	–	<3.4[d]

[a] Attempts should also be made to increase HDL-C and lower triglyceride levels in appropriate patients.
[b] Optional if low-density lipoprotein cholesterol <2.6 mmol/L.
[c] Targets should be individualised to each patient and the calculated risk.
[d] if TG ≥3.4 mmol/L.

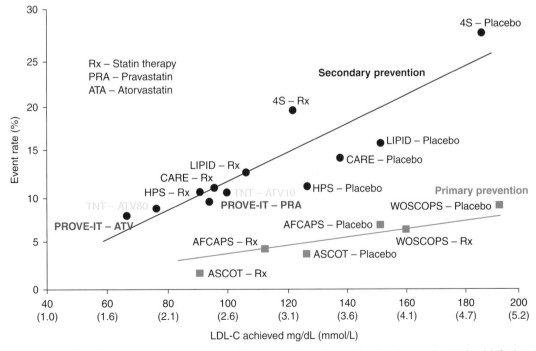

Figure 8.3 Achieving lower LDL-C reduces coronary events. The data show that lower LDL-C levels reduce cardiovascular risk further, therefore supporting the concept that the lower you can get your LDL-C the better. *Source*: Adapted with permission from a figure published in Ref. 17. Copyright Elsevier (1998).

Table 8.5 Primary and secondary lipid targets

Cholesterol guidelines	Primary lipid goal	Secondary goal
Australia	TC	–
Canada	LDL-C	TC: HDL-C ratio
Europe	LDL-C or TC	–
New Zealand	LDL-C or TC	TC: HDL-C ratio
United States	LDL-C	Non-HDL-C
International	LDL-C	Non-HDL-C

TC: Total cholesterol.

pharmacotherapy can cause adverse effects and should be monitored appropriately.

The first follow-up visit should occur 6–12 weeks after initiating drug therapy, by which stage the maximal treatment effect will have occurred. In the case of nicotinic acid, where doses must be titrated by the patient to a therapeutic level, the first follow-up visit should occur 6–12 weeks after the patient has reached the initial targeted dose. If the initial dose of the drug must be increased or another drug added in order to reach the treatment goal, the patient should be seen in another 6–12 weeks for follow-up evaluation of the new drug regimen. This process should be repeated until the patient has reached the treatment goal. Repeated monitoring of CK and liver enzymes is more controversial since routinely measured CK will not detect rhabdomyolysis and liver function tests may vary for many reasons in free living individuals. However, rises in liver enzymes will occur more frequently as doses of statin are up-titrated and may prevent such titrations.

Once the patient has achieved the treatment goal, follow-up intervals may be reduced to every 4–6 months. Lipoprotein profiles should be assessed at least annually. Follow-up visits can be used to enhance adherence and to determine whether persons have achieved their treatment goal. If they have not, changes in the drug regimen can be made to attempt to reach these goals. Several studies have investigated the effect of strategies to maximise adherence with lipid-modifying therapy on subsequent lipid levels (see long-term management of cardiovascular disease section).

Conclusion

Pharmacological treatment is warranted in patients unable to achieve lipid goals with lifestyle changes, and has been shown to have a significant impact on cardiovascular outcomes. An LDL-C level below 2.6 mmol/L is the primary goal in high-risk patients, and recent trials support the benefit of achieving this goal, or even lower levels.

Table 8.6 Monitoring and follow-up of lipid-lowering therapies

Drug	Monitoring parameters	Follow-up schedule
Bile acid sequestrants	Indigestion, bloating, constipation, abdominal pain, flatulence, nausea	Evaluate symptoms initially and at each follow-up visit
		Also check time of administration with other drugs
Nicotinic Acid	Flushing, itching, tingling, headache, nausea, gas, heartburn, fatigue, rash	Evaluate symptoms initially and at each follow-up visit
	Peptic ulcer	Evaluate symptoms initially, then as needed
	Fasting blood sugar (FBS)	Obtain an FBS and uric acid initially, 6–8 weeks after starting therapy, then annually or more frequently if indicated to monitor for hyperglycaemia and hyperuricaemia
	Uric acid	
	ALT and AST	Obtain an ALT/AST initially after reaching a daily dose of 1,500 mg, 6–8 weeks after reaching the maximum daily dose, then annually or more frequently if indicated
Statins	Muscle soreness, tenderness or pain	Evaluate muscle symptoms initially. Evaluate muscle symptoms at each follow-up visit. Obtain a CK when persons have muscle soreness, tenderness or pain
	ALT, AST	Evaluate ALT/AST initially, approximately 12 weeks after starting, then annually or more frequently if indicated
Fibrates	Abdominal pain, dyspepsia, headache, drowsiness	Evaluate symptoms initially and at each follow-up visit
	Cholelithiasis	Evaluate history and symptoms initially and then as needed

CK, Creatine kinase; ALT, alanine aminotransferase; AST, aspartate aminotransferase.

 Source: Third Report of the National Cholesterol Education Program (2001) produced by the NHLBI (part of the NIH and the US Department of Health & Human Services. Available at: http://www.nhlbi.nih.gov/guidelines/cholesterol/index.htm

References

1. Prevention of cardiovascular disease: An evidence-based clinical aid. *Med J Aust.* 2004; 181: F1–1.
2. Genest J, Frohlich J, Fodor G, McPherson R. Recommendations for the management of dyslipidemia and the prevention of cardiovascular disease: 2003 update. *CMAJ.* 2003; 169: 921–4.
3. Graham I, Atar AE, Borch-Johsen K et al. European guidelines on cardiovascular disease prevention in clinical practice. *Eur J Cardiovasc Prev Rehabil.* 2007; 14(Suppl 2): S1–113.
4. The assessment and management of cardiovascular risk. Available at http://www.nzgg.org.nz/index.cfm?fuseaction=fuseaction_10&fusesubaction=docs&documentid=22 (Accessed October 2007).
5. Third report of the National Cholesterol Education Program (NCEP) expert panel on detection, evaluation, and treatment of high blood cholesterol in adults (Adult Treatment Panel III) (2001). Expert panel on detection, evaluation, and treatment of high blood cholesterol in adults. *JAMA.* 2001; 285: 2486–97.
6. Grundy SM, Cleeman JI, Bairey CN et al. Implications of Recent Clinical Trials for the National Cholesterol Education Program Adult Treatment Panel III Guidelines – 2004 update. *Circulation.* 2004; 110: 227–39.
7. International Atherosclerosis Society (IAS) (2003). Harmonized guidelines on prevention of atherosclerotic cardiovascular diseases. Available at http://www.athero.org/ (Accessed October 2007).
8. Gould AL, Rossouw JE, Santanello NC et al. Cholesterol reduction yields clinical benefit: Impact of statin trials. *Circ.* 1998; 97: 946–52.
9. Studer M. Effect of different antilipidemic agents and diets on mortality: A systematic review. *Arch Intern Med.* 2005; 165(7): 725–30.
10. Grundy SM. The issue of statin safety: where do we stand? *Circ.* 2005; 111(23): 3016–9.
11. Jones PH. Comparison of the efficacy and safety of rosuvastatin versus atorvastatin, simvastatin, and pravastatin across doses (STELLAR* Trial). *Am J Cardiol.* 2003 July 15; 92(2): 152–60.
12. Keech A, Simes RJ, Barter P et al, for the FIELD Study investigators. Effects of long term fenofibrate therapy on cardiovascular events in 9n795 people with type 2 idabetes mellitus (the FIELD Study): Randomised controlled trial. Lancet 2005;366:1849–1861.
13. Pearson TA. A community-based, randomized trial of ezetimibe added to statin therapy to attain NCEP ATP III goals for LDL cholesterol in hypercholesterolemic patients: The ezetimibe add-on to statin for effectiveness (EASE) trial. *Mayo Clin Proc.* 2005; 80(5): 587–95.
14. Kastelein JJP, Akdim F, Stroes ESJ et al for the ENHANCE investigators. Simvastatin with or without Ezetimibe in Familial Hypercholesterolemia. *New Engl J Med.* 2008;358:1431–1443.
15. Cannon CP et al. Intensive versus moderate lipid lowering with statins after acute coronary syndromes. *N Engl J Med.* 2004; 350(15): 1495–504.
16. LaRosa JC. Intensive lipid lowering with atorvastatin in patients with stable coronary disease. *N Engl J Med.* 2005; 352(14): 1425–35.
17. Ballantyne CM. Low-density lipoproteins and risk for coronary heart disease. *Am J Cardiol.* 1998; 82(9A): 3Q–12Q.

9

Pharmacotherapy: lowering blood pressure

B. Arroll[1], A. Fitton[2] and S. Mann[3]

[1]University of Auckland, Auckland, New Zealand
[2]The Future Forum Secretariat, London, UK
[3]University of Otago, Wellington Clinical School, Wellington, New Zealand

Introduction

Elevated blood pressure is a major risk factor for stroke, coronary artery disease, congestive heart failure and renal failure, and management of hypertension is a vital component of cardiovascular risk reduction strategies. However, notwithstanding the widespread availability of cardiovascular disease (CVD) prevention guidelines (Box 9.1)[1-7] and hypertension management guidelines (Box 9.2),[8-11] hypertension remains suboptimally managed, even in affluent 'first world' countries, and many patients remain at unnecessarily increased cardiovascular risk. For example, in the United States, it is estimated that only 50% of patients with hypertension receive treatment, and fewer than 30% have adequately controlled blood pressure. Some of this can be explained by clinician and patient factors as well as the lack of blood pressure lowering capacity of most current antihypertensive medications. Many patients require more than one medication to reach target levels and this can create difficulties in terms of adherence. In those patients with isolated systolic hypertension, blood pressure lowering can be very difficult even with multiple medications. This is significant as this group of patients is likely to rise with the increase in elderly patients in most developed countries.

Who gets high blood pressure?

Apart from genetic predisposition (it is estimated that 30–60% of cases of essential hypertension are inherited), non-modifiable risk factors for hypertension include advancing age, ethnicity, low-birth weight and seasonal influences. Circadian and seasonal variations in blood pressure can be substantial, and these

Box 9.1 Regional and national guidelines for prevention of CVD

 Australia: Practical Implementation Taskforce for the Prevention of CVD (2004)
http://www.mja.com.au/public/issues/181_06_200904/ful10382_fm.html

 Canada: Working Group on Hypercholesterolemia and Other Dyslipidemias (2003)
http://www.cmaj.ca/cgi/content/full/169/9/921/DC1

 Europe: Third Joint European Task Force (2007)
http://www.escardio.org/knowledge/guidelines/CVD_Prevention_in_Clinical_Practice.htm

 New Zealand: New Zealand Guidelines Group, NHF and Stroke Foundation (2003)
http://www.nzgg.org.nz/index.cfm?fuseaction=fuseaction_10&fusesubaction=docs&documentid=22

 United States: Third Report of the National Cholesterol Education Program (2001, 2004)
http://jama.ama-assn.org/cgi/content/full/285/19/2486
http://www.nhlbi.n`ih.gov/guidelines/cholesterol/atp3upd04.pdf

 International: International Atherosclerosis Society (2003)
http://www.athero.org/

temporal effects should be considered when diagnosing and treating hypertension (Figures 9.1 and 9.2).[12,13] Blood pressure has been falling among younger people for the past few decades. This is largely unexplained and it is not clear how the looming obesity epidemic will counter this. Among the modifiable risk factors for hypertension, obesity, unhealthy diet (high sodium and alcohol intake), a sedentary lifestyle and mental stress are major influences. As an illustration of the apparent effect of lifestyle on hypertensive risk, the Yanomamo

Box 9.2 National and international guidelines for treatment of hypertension

 Europe: Guidelines Committee. 2003 European Society of Hypertension – European Society of Cardiology guidelines for the management of arterial hypertension. *J Hypertens*. 2003; 21: 1011–53.
http://www.eshonline.org/ documents/2003_guidelines.pdf

 United Kingdom: British Hypertension Society guidelines for hypertension management 2004 (BHS-IV): Summary. *BMJ*. 2004; 328: 634–640.
http://bmj.bmjjournals.com/cgi/content/full/328/7440/634

 United States: Seventh report of the Joint National Committee on prevention, detection, evaluation, and treatment of high blood pressure. *Hypertension*. 2003; 42: 1206–52.
http://hyper.ahajournals.org/cgi/content/full/42/6/1206

 International: 2003 World Health Organization (WHO)/International Society of Hypertension (ISH) statement on management of hypertension. *J Hypertens*. 2003; 21: 1983–92.

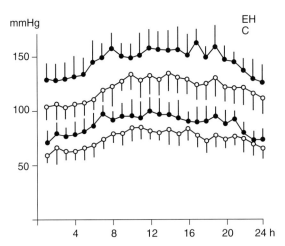

Figure 9.1 Mean (±SE) 24-hour blood pressure profiles of normotensive (○) and untreated hypertensive (●) patients. *Source*: Reproduced from Ref. 12.

Indians of the Amazon, who subsist on a diet very low in salt (<0.5 g/day) and saturated fats, do not smoke, and lead physically active lives, have low blood pressures (mean 96/60 mmHg; range 78/37 to 128/86 mmHg) throughout adulthood, with no age-related rise beyond the second decade of life, and experience little or no hypertension or vascular disease

(Figure 9.3). However, when they adopt a western lifestyle, they become overweight, and susceptible to diabetes and premature vascular disease.[15] Such evidence indicates that hypertension could theoretically be prevented if western society changed its diet and lifestyle, but such extreme lifestyle changes are probably not feasible.

Blood pressure and cardiovascular risk

Hypertension is usually defined as a blood pressure ≥140/90 mmHg. However, there is a continuous graded relationship between blood pressure and CVD risk (Figure 9.4),[16] and blood-pressure-lowering is beneficial for all hypertensive categories.[17] Long-term reductions in systolic and diastolic blood pressures of 10–12 and 56 mmHg, respectively, have been shown to produce a 35–40% reduction in the risk of stroke and a 20–25% reduction in the risk of coronary heart disease in patients with mild-to-moderate hypertension.

Target blood pressures for hypertensive patients are inversely related to cardiovascular risk. For individuals at low-to-moderate risk, a blood pressure goal of <140/90 mmHg is usually recommended; for individuals at higher risk, the blood pressure target may vary between 140/90 and 130/80 mmHg, depending on level of risk and physician preference. Patients with diabetes and hypertension are at particularly high risk, and target blood pressures of 130/85 or 130/80 mmHg are usually recommended for this population. Lower targets, such as a diastolic level of 75 mmHg, may be indicated in individuals with diabetes and concurrent renal disease.

When is drug treatment required?

Determination of the need for drug therapy is based on the absolute risk of CVD, which is governed by blood pressure level, coexistent risk factors and the presence/absence of hypertensive end-organ damage (Box 9.3). For patients at low-to-moderate risk, initial attempts to control hypertension should be based on lifestyle changes, including weight reduction, dietary modification (salt and alcohol restriction) and promotion of physical exercise. If this approach proves ineffective or if blood pressure is considerably elevated, antihypertensive medication should be introduced. That degree of blood pressure elevation differs from country to country, ranging from >140/90 mmHg according to the World Health Organization/International Society of Hypertension guidelines to >170/100 mmHg according to the New Zealand guidelines.[4,11] For diabetic patients and those with multiple cardiovascular risk factors or target-organ (cerebrovascular, cardiac, renal or retinal) disease, pharmacological and non-pharmacological measures are usually instituted simultaneously.

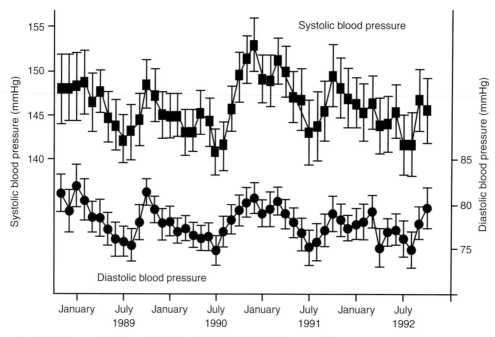

Figure 9.2 Seasonal variation in mean (±SE) systolic (■) and diastolic (●) blood pressures in a French study of haemodialysis patients with end-stage renal disease. *Source*: Reproduced with permission. Copyright [1998] Massachusetts Medical Society. All rights reserved. Ref. 13.

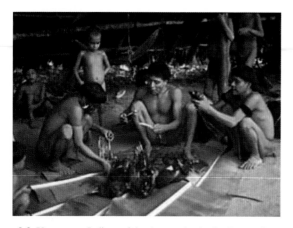

Figure 9.3 Yanomamo Indians of the Amazonian basin. *Source*: Image reproduced with permission from Napoleon A. Chagnon. Ref. 14.

Pharmacological management of hypertension

It is important that any antihypertensive medication has a favourable safety profile and is effective in reducing cardiovascular morbidity and mortality. Five drug classes satisfy these criteria: diuretics, beta-blockers, angiotensin converting-enzyme inhibitors (ACEIs), angiotensin II receptor antagonists (ARBs) and calcium channel blockers.[18–20] It should be noted that short-acting calcium channel blockers are not recommended for management of hypertension because they are associated

with increased risks of myocardial infarction (MI) and cardiovascular mortality.

In general, the benefits of antihypertensive treatment are related to the magnitude of reduction in blood pressure.[20] For some disease conditions, however, particular antihypertensive drug classes may be associated with superior outcomes that are independent of their antihypertensive effect. Conversely, some classes of drug are contraindicated in patients with particular disease conditions. Thus, the choice of antihypertensive medication may be influenced by patient comorbidity. It should be noted that, for many patients, a combination of two or more antihypertensive agents selected from different drug classes is required to achieve adequate blood pressure control. Consequently, the task is to determine the best treatment regimen rather than the best initial agent.

Hypertensive patients without specific comorbidities

For hypertensive patients without specific comorbidities, thiazide diuretics are widely recommended as initial therapy, although ACEIs, ARBs, beta-blockers and calcium channel blockers are also suitable. Patient age and ethnic background may dictate the preferred class of drug, but it should be emphasised that choice of agent is far less important than ensuring that target blood pressure goals are met. Thiazide diuretics and beta-blockers have a poor image because of their potentially detrimental effects on glycaemic control, but both these drug classes (apart from atenonol, which is under a cloud at present)

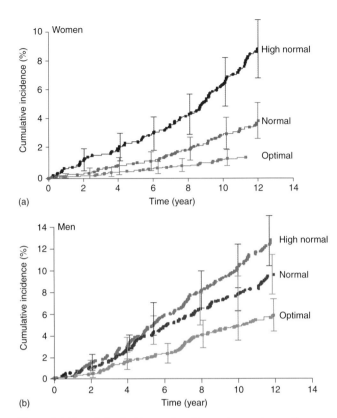

(a)

(b)

Figure 9.4 Cumulative incidence of cardiovascular events over time in non-hypertensive women (A) and men (B) categorized according to their blood pressure at baseline examination. Vertical bars indicate 95% CI. Blood pressure was defined as 'optimal' (<120/<80 mmHg), 'normal' (120–129 or 80–84 mmHg), or 'high-normal' (130–139 or 85–89 mmHg). *Source*: Reproduced with permission. Copyright © [2001] Massachusetts Medical Society. All rights reserved. Ref. 16.

Box 9.3 Cardiovascular risk factors

- **Major risk factors**
  - Hypertension
  - Obesity (BMI ≥30 kg/m²)
  - Cigarette smoking
  - Dyslipidaemia
  - Physical inactivity
  - Diabetes mellitus
  - Microalbuminuria
  - Family history of premature CVD
  - Age (men >55 years; women >65 years)

- **Target-organ damage**
  - Left ventricular hypertrophy
  - Heart failure
  - Angina or prior myocardial infarction
  - Prior coronary revascularization
  - Stroke/TIA
  - Peripheral arterial disease
  - Chronic renal disease
  - Retinopathy.

Table 9.1 Treatment of hypertensive patients with a history of cardiac disease

BP goal:	• All patients, 130/80–140/90 mmHg	
Drug class	Compelling indication	Comments
ACEI	✓	} Reduce cardiovascular
β-blocker	✓	} morbidity and mortality

have been shown to be highly effective in reducing cardiovascular morbidity and mortality in hypertensive patients.

In regard to the best initial agent (especially in older patients), there has been a concern that beta blockers (mainly atenolol) may offer poorer blood pressure reduction and less protection against stroke and myocardial infarction than other agents.[21,22] Another recent large systematic review has however suggested that all classes of antihypertensive agents were equally effective in terms of cardiovascular outcomes in both old and young patients.[23] Older patients will generally get more immediate benefit from therapy given their higher absolute risk.[23]

The AB/CD rule outlined in the UK guidelines is a reasonable approach to lowering blood pressure but is not based on significant clinical outcomes such as death or CVD.[9] The guideline states 'The theory underpinning the AB/CD algorithm is that hypertension can be broadly classified as "high renin" or "low rennin" and is therefore best treated initially with one of two categories of antihypertensive drug – those that inhibit the renin–angiotensin system (ACEIs/ARBs [A] or beta-blockers [B]), and those that do not (calcium channel blockers [C] or diuretics [D]). People who are younger than 55 and white (Caucasian) tend to have higher renin concentrations than people aged 55 or older, or of African descent. A or B drugs are therefore generally more effective as initial blood pressure-lowering treatment in younger white patients than C or D drugs. However, C or D drugs are more effective first-line agents for older white people or people of African descent of any age. When the first drug is well tolerated but the response is small and insufficient, substitution of an alternative drug is appropriate if hypertension is mild and uncomplicated. In more severe or complicated hypertension it is safer to add drugs stepwise until blood pressure is controlled. Treatment can be stepped down later if blood pressure falls substantially below the optimal level.

Patients with a history of myocardial infarction

Beta-blockers and ACEIs are of established benefit in reducing cardiovascular morbidity and mortality in patients with a history of MI and are the preferred antihypertensive drugs for use in this population, either as monotherapy or in combination (Table 9.1). It should be noted that ACEIs are particularly indicated in patients with left ventricular dysfunction or heart failure (Table 9.2). Evidence for the benefit of calcium channel blockers in acute MI is equivocal and these agents should

Table 9.2 Treatment of hypertensive patients with heart failure

BP goal:	• Not firmly established • SBP <100 mmHg may be beneficial in some patients	
Drug class	Compelling indication	Comments
ACEI	✓	Reduce risk of mortality in patients at high risk of CVD
ARB		Indicated in patients intolerant of ACEIs
β-blocker	✓	Indicated in combination with ACEIs for patients with NYHA class II, III and IV heart failure
Diuretic (thiazides)		May prevent disease progression
CCB (rate-limiting)		*Contraindicated*; may further depress cardiac function

Table 9.3 Use of antihypertensive drugs for secondary stroke prevention

BP goal:	• Treatment indicated in all normotensive and hypertensive post-stroke patients	
Drug class	Compelling indication	Comments
ACEI **Diuretic (thiazide or thiazide-like)**	✓ ✓	} Particularly effective in preventing recurrent stroke when used in combination

not be used as first-line therapy for treating hypertension in the post-MI setting. Immediate-release nifedipine is contraindicated in patients with acute MI, and immediate-release verapamil should be avoided in patients with left ventricular dysfunction. There is no clear consensus as to whether antihypertensive drugs should be prescribed for all post-MI patients, or only for those with hypertension.

Patients with a history of stroke or transient ischaemic attack

For patients with cerebrovascular disease, blood pressure is a determinant of stroke risk among both hypertensive and non-hypertensive individuals.[24] Thus, blood pressure should be lowered in all non-hypotensive patients who have survived a stroke or transient ischaemic attack (TIA). Thiazide diuretics and ACEIs are the preferred drug classes in this patient group (Table 9.3), and appear to be particularly effective in reducing the risk of recurrent stroke and major vascular events when used in combination.

Patients with diabetes or prediabetes

Diabetic individuals require aggressive control of blood pressure, and combination therapy is frequently necessary. For patients without concurrent renal disease, ACEIs, ARBs, thiazide diuretics, beta-blockers and calcium channel blockers are all appropriate (Table 9.4). For diabetic patients with renal disease, an ACEI or an ARB should be included in the antihypertensive regimen on account of their nephroprotective properties. ACEIs are preferred for patients with concurrent microalbuminuria, type I diabetic nephropathy or other renal disease, whereas ARBs are indicated in patients with Type 2 diabetic nephropathy and in those who are intolerant of ACEIs.

Table 9.4 Treatment of hypertensive diabetic patients*

BP goal:	• No renal disease: 130/80–130/85 mmHg • Concurrent renal disease: <130/80 mmHg • Proteinuria: diastolic BP 75 mmHg		
Comorbidity	Drug class	Compelling indication	Comments
None	**ACEI**		Particularly recommended for CVD prevention in high-risk patients; more effective when used in combination therapy
	ARB		
	Thiazides		Tendency to worsen hyperglycaemia but effect is slight and generally clinically insignificant
	β-blocker		
CVD	**β-blocker**	✓	} Consider using in combination
	ACEI	✓	
DN (Type 1 diabetes)	**ACEI**	✓	} Delay deterioration in renal function
Microalbuminuria	**ACEI ± ARB**	✓	
DN (Type 2 diabetes)	**ARB**	✓	

*The majority of diabetic patients require combination therapy with at least 2 antihypertensive agents to achieve adequate control of blood pressure.

Table 9.5 Treatment of hypertensive non-diabetic patients with renal disease*

BP goal:	• 130/80 mmHg		
Renal pathology	Drug class	Possible indications	Comments
Chronic renal disease	**Diuretic**		Should be used in combination with ACEI/ARB therapy; loop diuretics generally preferred to thiazide diuretics
	ACEI	✓	⎱ Limit progression of chronic renal disease, but should be used with
	ARB	✓	⎰ caution in patients with significant renal impairment
Proteinuria	**ACEI**	✓	
	ARB	✓	
Renovascular disease	**ACEI**		⎱ Generally *contraindicated*, but may be used under specialist
	ARB		⎰ supervision**

*The majority of patients with chronic renal disease require combination therapy with at least two antihypertensive agents to achieve adequate blood pressure control.
**Serum creatinine should be checked on initiating ACEI or ARB therapy if renal artery stenosis is suspected.

Table 9.6 Treatment of isolated systolic hypertension in elderly patients

BP goal:	• 140/90 mmHg		
Drug class	Compelling indication	May be used	Comments
CCB (dihydropyridine)	✓		Choice of agent less important than degree of BP reduction achieved; adequate control of BP reduces risk of all CV events, including stroke
Diuretic (thiazide or thiazide-like)	✓		
ACEI		✓	
ARB		✓	
B-blocker		✓	

Key to Tables 1–6:

Indicated

Use with caution

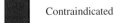

Contraindicated

ACEI, angiotensin converting enzyme inhibitor; ARB, angiotension II receptor blocker; BP, blood pressure; CCB, calcium channel blocker; CV, cardiovascular; CVD, cardiovascular disease; DN, diabetic nephropathy; ISH, isolated systolic hypertension; SBP, systolic blood pressure; TIA, transient ischaemic attack.

Diabetic patients with a history of CVD may benefit from combination therapy with an ACEI and a beta-blocker.

The first choice antihypertensive therapies in patients with prediabetes (i.e. impaired glucose tolerance and impaired fasting glucose) is unclear as there is concern about the diabetogenic potential of diuretics and beta-blockers in some patients.

Non-diabetic patients with renal disease

ACEIs and ARBs are more effective than other drug classes at slowing progression of chronic renal disease. For this reason, a drug from one of these classes should be included in the antihypertensive regimen of all non-diabetic patients with renal disease

(Table 9.5). Many patients will require combination therapy, in which case the ACEI/ARB can be used in conjunction with a diuretic. Loop diuretics, rather than thiazides, will be required by many patients with elevated serum creatinine levels. Although chronic renal disease is a compelling indication for use of an ACEI or an ARB, these drugs should be used with caution in patients with significant renal impairment. Furthermore, these drug classes are specifically contraindicated in patients with renovascular disease. Serum creatinine levels should be measured shortly after initiating ACEI or ARB therapy; several authorities suggest that an increase of up to 25% is acceptable, but ongoing monitoring is essential in such cases.

Elderly patients

Isolated systolic hypertension, which is common in the elderly, is associated with increased risk of stroke and other occlusive events. Aggressive antihypertensive management is effective in reducing cardiovascular risk and is thus indicated in this population. Thiazide diuretics are usually the drug of first choice; their use in the elderly should be accompanied by monitoring of electrolyte levels (Table 9.6). If thiazides cannot be tolerated, long-acting dihydropyridine calcium channel blockers are a suitable alternative. Beta-blockers, ACEIs and ARBs are also suitable for elderly hypertensive patients.

Conclusions

It is important to recognise that the positive relationship between blood pressure and cardiovascular risk commences at blood pressures substantially lower than the commonly accepted definition of hypertension. For example, it has been estimated that each 20/10 mmHg increment above a baseline pressure of 115/75 mmHg is associated with a doubling of cardiovascular risk in individuals aged 40–70 years.

Thiazide diuretics have shown good efficacy in clinical trials and are relatively inexpensive; for this reason they are frequently used as the basis of treatment in patients with uncomplicated hypertension. The AB/CD algorithm in the UK guidelines provides a more detailed approach to initial treatment. For patients with specific comorbidities, other drug classes may be indicated. It should be recognised that monotherapy is usually inadequate for patients with high-risk conditions (e.g. diabetes, chronic renal disease) and low blood-pressure goals, and two or more antihypertensive medications are generally required for adequate control of blood pressure in these patients.

References

1. Prevention of cardiovascular disease: An evidence-based clinical aid. *Med J Aust.* 2004; 181: F1–14.
2. Genest J, Frohlich J, Fodor G et al. Recommendations for the management of dyslipidemia and the prevention of cardiovascular disease: 2003 update. *CMAJ.* 2003; 169: 921–4.
3. Graham I, Atar AE, Borch-Johnsen K et al. European guidelines on cardiovascular disease prevention in clinical practice. *Eur J Cardiovasc Prev Rehabil.* 2007; 14(Suppl 2): S1–113.
4. The assessment and management of cardiovascular risk. Available at http://www.nzgg.org.nz/index.cfm?fuseaction=fuseaction_10& fusesubaction=docs&documentid=22 (Accessed October 2007).
5. Third report of the National Cholesterol Education Program (NCEP) expert panel on detection, evaluation, and treatment of high blood cholesterol in adults (Adult Treatment Panel III) (2001). Expert panel on detection, evaluation, and treatment of high blood cholesterol in adults. *JAMA.* 2001; 285: 2486–97.
6. Grundy SM, Cleeman JI, Bairey CN et al. Implications of recent clinical trials for the national cholesterol education program adult treatment panel III guidelines – 2004 update. *Circulation.* 2004; 110: 227–39.
7. International Atherosclerosis Society (IAS) (2003). Harmonized guidelines on prevention of atherosclerotic cardiovascular diseases. Available at http://www.athero.org/ (Accessed October 2007).
8. European Society of Cardiology guidelines for the management of arterial hypertension. *J Hypertens.* 2003; 21: 1011–53.
9. British Hypertension Society guidelines for hypertension management 2004 (BHS-IV): Summary. *BMJ.* 2004; 328: 634–40.
10. Seventh report of the Joint National Committee on prevention, detection, evaluation, and treatment of high blood pressure. *Hypertension.* 2003; 42: 1206–52.
11. 2003 World Health Organization (WHO)/International Society of Hypertension (ISH) statement on management of hypertension. *J Hypertens.* 2003; 21: 1983–92.
12. Siegelová J, Fiser B, Dusek J et al. Circadian variability of rate-pressure product in essential hypertension with enlapril therapy. *Scripta Medica (Brno).* 2000; 73: 67–75.
13. Argilés A, Mourad G, Mion C. Seasonal changes in blood pressure in patients with end-stage renal disease treated with hemodialysis. *NEJM.* 1998; 339: 1364–70.
14. Napoleon A. Chagnon. http://www.anth.ucsb.edu/projects/axfight/gallery.html (Accessed October 2007).
15. Mancilha-Carvalho JJ, de Oliveira R, Esposito RJ. Blood pressure and electrolyte excretion in the Yanomamo Indians, an isolated population. *J Hum Hypertens.* 1989; 3: 309–14.
16. Vasan RS, Larson MG, Leip EP et al. Impact of high-normal blood pressure on the risk of cardiovascular disease. *N Engl J Med.* 2001; 345: 1291–7.
17. MacMahon S, Peto R, Cutler J et al. Blood pressure, stroke, and coronary heart disease. Part 1. Prolonged differences in blood pressure: Prospective observational studies corrected for the regression dilution bias. *Lancet.* 1990; 335: 765–74.
18. Foody JM, Farrell MH, Krumholz HM. Beta-blocker therapy in heart failure: Scientific review. *J Am Med Assoc.* 2002; 287: 883–9.
19. Neal B, MacMahon S, Chapman N, for the Blood Pressure Lowering Treatment Trialists' Collaboration. Effects of ACE inhibitors, calcium antagonists, and other blood-pressure-lowering drugs: Results of prospectively designed overviews of randomised trials. *Lancet.* 2000; 356: 1955–64.
20. Turnbull F, for the Blood Pressure Lowering Treatment Trialists' Collaboration. Effects of different blood-pressure-lowering regimens on major cardiovascular events: Results of prospectively-designed overviews of randomised trials. *Lancet.* 2003; 362: 1527–35.
21. Beevers DG. The end of B(eta) blockers for uncomplicated hypertension. Lancet 2005; 336:1511–2.
22. Wiysonge CS, Bradley H, Mayosi BM, Maroney R, Mbewu A, Opie LH, Volmink J. Beta-blockers for hypertension. *Cochrane Database of Systematic Reviews* 2007, Issue 1. Art. No.: CD002003. DOI: 10.1002/14651858.CD002003.pub2.
23. Blood pressure lowering treatment trialists collaboration. Effects of different regiments to lower blood pressure on major cardiovascular events in older and younger adults: meta-analysis of randomized trials. BMJ 2008 doi:10.1136/bmj.39548.738368.BE (published 14 May 2008).
24. Collins R, Peto R, MacMahon S et al. Blood pressure, stroke, and coronary heart disease. Part 2. Short-term reductions in blood pressure: Overview of randomised drug trials in their epidemiological context. *Lancet.* 1990; 335: 827–38.

10 Pharmacotherapy: lowering blood glucose

T. Kenealy[1], A. Fitton[2] and L.A. Leiter[3]

[1]University of Auckland, Auckland, New Zealand
[2]The Future Forum Secretariat, London, UK
[3]University of Toronto, Toronto, Canada

Introduction

Both type 1 and type 2 diabetes are characterised by hyperglycaemia and associated metabolic derangement that are associated with increased risk of morbidity and mortality. In type 1 diabetes, hyperglycaemia results from insulin deficiency caused by pancreatic beta-cell destruction. In contrast, the hyperglycaemia of type 2 diabetes results from a combination of insulin resistance and defective insulin secretion. Glycaemic control can be assessed by measuring fasting and post-prandial plasma glucose levels, and by determining the plasma level of glycosylated haemoglobin (HbA_{1c}), which positively correlates with the average plasma glucose level over the preceding 2–3 months (Table 10.1).[1]

It is well established that tight control of blood glucose delays the onset and slows the progression of microvascular complications in both type 1 and type 2 diabetes.[2,3] Long-term follow-up of patients in the Diabetes Control and Complications Trial indicated that intensive glucose control in type 1 diabetes was associated with a 42% reduction in risk of cardiovascular events and a 57% reduction in risk of non-fatal myocardial infarction, stroke or death from cardiovascular disease.[4,5] Although the effects of optimal blood glucose control on macrovascular risk are less clear, particularly in type 2 diabetes, reductions in HbA_{1c} have been associated with reduced risk of myocardial infarction, stroke, heart failure and diabetes-related mortality.[6] The relationship between HbA_{1c} level and cardiovascular risk is continuous, and there is no evidence that there is a threshold HbA_{1c} level below which risk does not decrease. Consequently, tight control of blood glucose levels is strongly recommended in all diabetes management guidelines. In general, the means by which normal glucose levels are

Table 10.1 Relationship between HbA_{1c} level and mean plasma glucose level in type 1 diabetes

HbA_{1c} (%)	Mean plasma glucose	
	mmol/L	mg/dL
6	7.5	135
7	9.5	170
8	11.5	205
9	13.5	240
10	15.5	275
11	17.5	310
12	19.5	345

Copyright © 2002 American Diabetes Association. Reprinted with permission from The American Diabetes Association. *Source*: Ref. 1.

attained are less important than ensuring that the target levels are reached. The recommendations for management of blood glucose made in this article are taken from current guidelines (Box 10.1).[7–10]

The role of lifestyle

Lifestyle plays an important role in the management of type 1 and type 2 diabetes. Dietary control and physical activity are important therapeutic tools that can substantially reduce plasma glucose levels and, in type 2 diabetes, can reduce peripheral insulin resistance (thereby benefiting not only glucose but also blood pressure and lipids). However, in type 2 diabetes optimal lifestyle modification alone is often insufficient to maintain HbA_{1c} below target levels (Table 10.2), and it is generally recommended that pharmacological intervention should be initiated either from diagnosis or certainly if lifestyle changes fail to achieve glycaemic targets within 2–3 months. For patients

Cardiovascular Risk Management, Edited by R Hobbs and B Arroll
© 2009 Blackwell Publishing, ISBN: 9781405155755

Box 10.1 Guidelines for management of patients with diabetes

American Diabetes Association (2007)
2007 Clinical Practice Recommendations. Standards of Medical Care in Diabetes
Diabetes Care. 2007; 30 (Suppl 1): S3–103
http://www.diabetes.org/for-health-professionals-and-scientists/cpr.jsp

- Summary of current American Diabetes Association recommendations for the management of patients with diabetes
- Includes sections on diagnosis, screening, evaluation, glycaemic control, physical activity and prevention and management of complications
- Updated annually

American Association of Clinical Endocrinologists (2007)
Medical guidelines for the management of diabetes mellitus
Endocr Pract. 2007; 13 (Suppl 1): 1–68
http://www.aace.com/pub/pdf/guidelines/DMGuidelines2007.pdf

- Outlines a systematic multidisciplinary approach to the management of diabetes that aims to help physicians to provide intensive therapy for patients with diabetes
- Emphasises active patient participation in the management of the disease

Canadian Diabetes Association Clinical Practice Guidelines Expert Committee (2003)
Clinical Practice Guidelines for the Prevention and Management of Diabetes in Canada
Can J Diabetes. 2003; 27 (Suppl 2): S1–152
http://www.diabetes.ca/cpg2003/default.aspx

- Comprehensive, current guidelines on the management of diabetes
- Includes chapters on targets for glycaemic control and on pharmacological management of hyperglycaemia

American Diabetes Association and the European Association for the Study of Diabetes (2006)
Management of hyperglycaemia in type 2 diabetes: a consensus algorithm for the initiation and adjustment of therapy
Diabetologia. 2006; 49: 1711–21
http://www.springerlink.com/content/24j1675h2p72636v/fulltext.pdf

- Consensus approach to the treatment of hyperglycaemia in patients with type 2 diabetes
- Developed a treatment algorithm for the initiation and adjustment of therapy

International Diabetes Federation Clinical Guidelines Task Force (2005)
Global Guidelines for Type 2 Diabetes
Brussels: International Diabetes Federation, 2005
http://www.idf.org/home/index.cfm?node=1457

New Zealand Guidelines Group (2003)
Management of Type 2 Diabetes
http://www.nzgg.org.nz

- Comprehensive guidelines that include a lengthy, detailed section on all aspects of glycaemic control

with marked hyperglycaemia (e.g. HbA$_{1c}$ ≥ 9.0%), immediate pharmacological intervention in addition to lifestyle modification is usually warranted.[11]

The role of pharmacotherapy

For patients with type 1 diabetes, the primary pharmacological requirement is for exogenous insulin. In contrast, type 2 diabetes can be treated using a variety of agents (Box 10.2) that may be used alone or in combination to combat the abnormalities of glucose metabolism that characterise this disease. Thus, use of multiple drugs with complementary mechanisms of action may produce additive improvements in peripheral insulin resistance, hepatic insulin resistance (with excess glucose production) and impaired beta-cell function.

There is current controversy about how far to lower HbA$_{1c}$. The recent ACCORD trial reported an increase in deaths in a group targeting HbA$_{1c}$ of 6.0% or lower; they achieved a mean of 6.4%.[12] On the other hand the recent ADVANCE trial found no such increase in a group of apparently similar patients achieving the same HbA$_{1c}$.[13] The different results may be due to differences in the treatment regimens, but the controversy is unlikely to be resolved in the near future."

Table 10.2 Glycaemic targets for non-pregnant adults with diabetes

Parameter	Target	Comments
HbA$_{1c}$	⩽7.0%	A normal HbA$_{1c}$ target level (<6.0%) may be appropriate in selected patients*
		Low HbA$_{1c}$ target levels may be set for patients receiving only metformin or thiazolidinediones who are therefore at low risk of hypoglycaemia. Low HbA$_{1c}$ target levels are less advisable for patients receiving insulin or insulin secretagogues because of the associated risk of hypoglycaemia.
		A less stringent target (i.e. HbA$_{1c}$ > 7.0%) may be appropriate for • elderly patients • children • socially isolated patients • patients with limited life expectancy • patients with comorbid conditions • patients with hypoglycaemia unawareness
Preprandial plasma glucose	4.0–7.0 mmol/L (91–127 mg/dL)	A normal target range (4.0–6.0 mmol/L [73–109 mg/dL]) may be appropriate in selected patients* If HbA$_{1c}$ targets are not met, preprandial glucose levels should be targeted
Post-prandial plasma glucose	<10.0 mmol/L (<182 mg/dL)	Measurement should be made 1–2 hours after the beginning of the meal A normal target (<8.0 mmol/L [<145 mg/dL]) may be appropriate in selected patients* If preprandial glucose targets are met but HbA$_{1c}$ targets remain unmet, post-prandial glucose levels should be targeted

*Stringent glycaemic goals may reduce the risk of complications but increase the risk of hypoglycaemia
See text for discussion on target HbA$_{1c}$

Box 10.2 Pharmacological options for treatment of type 2 diabetes

Metformin
- *Primary effect*: Decreases hepatic glucose production
- *Secondary effect*: Decreases insulin resistance of muscle
- *Primary indication*: Patients with BMI > 25

Sulphonylureas (insulin secretagogues)
- *Primary effect*: Stimulate insulin secretion
- *Secondary effects*: Decrease hepatic glucose production, may improve insulin sensitivity
- *Primary indication*: Patients on metformin monotherapy who are not achieving glycaemic control (use in combination with metformin); thin patients with insulinopenia
- *Note*: Require functioning beta cells for activity

Meglitinides (insulin secretagogues)
- *Primary effect*: Stimulate release of insulin in response to rising plasma glucose levels, thereby lowering post-prandial plasma glucose levels
- *Secondary effect*: Reduce fasting plasma glucose levels
- *Primary indication*: Patients on metformin monotherapy who are not achieving glycaemic control (use in combination with metformin)
- *Note*: Require functioning beta cells for activity

α-Glucosidase inhibitors
- *Primary effect*: Inhibit α-glucosidase enzymes in small intestine, thereby delaying glucose absorption and reducing the post-prandial rise in plasma glucose levels
- *Secondary effect*: Lead to a small reduction in fasting plasma glucose levels
- *Primary indication*: Patients with exaggerated post-prandial hyperglycaemia

---

Box 10.2 *(Continued)*

Thiazolidinediones (insulin sensitisers)
- *Primary effect*: Decrease insulin resistance of peripheral muscle and fat cells
- *Secondary effect*: Decrease hepatic glucose production
- *Primary indication*: Patients with insulin resistance or impaired renal function (but not on dialysis)
- *Note*: Require the presence of insulin for activity

Dipeptidyl-peptidase 4 inhibitors
- *Primary effect*: Prolong the life of glucagon-like peptide-1 (GLP-1) to reduce post-prandial glucose excursions
- *Secondary effect*: Have a lesser effect on fasting plasma glucose
- *Primary indication*: As an adjunct to diet and exercise to improve glycaemic control in patients with type 2 diabetes mellitus

Insulin
- *Primary effects*: Decreases hepatic glucose production and increases peripheral glucose uptake
- *Primary indication*: Patients on maximum doses of oral agents in whom plasma glucose levels remain above goal, but can be used at any stage of type 2 diabetes
- *Note*: Inhaled insulin is now available in some countries for adult patients with type 1 and type 2 diabetes

---

Oral glucose-lowering agents

Oral glucose-lowering agents can be divided into four groups based on their mechanisms of action:

1. The biguanide, metformin, has been used as an antihyperglycaemic agent for more than 40 years. Metformin is believed to act primarily by suppressing the uncontrolled hepatic glucose production typically present in type 2 diabetes and by improving peripheral insulin sensitivity.

2. *Insulin secretagogues*: These comprise two main classes of drug – the sulphonylureas (e.g. glibenclamide, gliclazide, glipizide) and meglitinides (e.g. nateglinide, repaglinide), both of which require functional beta-cells for activity.

3. *Insulin sensitisers*: Increased insulin sensitivity is achieved by activation of the peroxisome proliferator-activated receptor-γ (PPAR-γ), which is the primary mode of action of the thiazolidinediones (e.g. pioglitazone, rosiglitazone).

4. α-Glucosidase inhibitors (e.g. acarbose) can be used to delay glucose absorption.

Some uncertainty has arisen about the role of rosiglitazone, and by implication perhaps other glitazones, following a recent meta-analysis that found an increase of cardiovascular deaths with this agent. The controversy is unlikely to be resolved soon.

Recently a new class of drugs has become available in some countries. These drugs augment activity of glucagon-like peptide-1 (GLP-1), a gastric hormone that stimulates glucose-dependent insulin secretion and insulin biosynthesis, and inhibits glucagon secretion, gastric emptying and food intake. These include exenatide, a GLP-1 agonist, and sitagliptin, a dipeptidyl-peptidase 4 inhibitor, which prolongs the half life of GLP-1.

For patients with type 2 diabetes, these oral agents may be used alone, in combination or in conjunction with insulin. The choice of treatment regimen is governed by clinical trial evidence, current and target HbA_{1c} levels, patient characteristics and physician preferences (Table 10.2). A treatment algorithm for management of hyperglycaemia, including oral agents and insulin, is shown in Figure 10.1. The main metabolic effects and therapeutic indications for these agents are shown in Box 10.2; the expected decreases in HbA_{1c} levels, the key contraindications to their use and the main adverse events associated with these agents are summarised in Tables 10.3, 10.4 and 10.5, respectively.

For overweight patients (body mass index $\geqslant 25\,kg/m^2$) with mild to moderate hyperglycaemia ($HbA_{1c} < 9.0\%$), metformin is the drug of first choice.[14] This biguanide has been shown to improve cardiovascular outcomes in this population, and it is one of the few antihyperglycaemic agents that are not associated with weight gain or hypoglycaemia. For patients who are not overweight, there is no compelling indication for metformin, and therapy can be initiated with various agents (Figure 10.1). For overweight patients with $HbA_{1c} > 9\%$, it is reasonable to initiate metformin, although it is likely that additional agents will be needed.

The patient's response after initiating therapy should be closely monitored. It should be remembered that, unlike the other drug classes, thiazolidinediones characteristically take several weeks to exert their effect, and that peak activity may not be evident for several months. For those patients who show inadequate reductions in plasma glucose levels, the treatment regimen should be intensified or supplemented with additional agents, with the aim of achieving target HbA_{1c} levels within 6 months of initial diagnosis. This may require frequent review of glucose results and subsequent adjustment of medication – making decisions only, for example, every 3 months, may mean that optimum control is delayed, sometimes indefinitely.

Insulin therapy in type 2 diabetes

Typically, glycaemic control shows progressive deterioration in patients with type 2 diabetes. Thus, with time there is a need

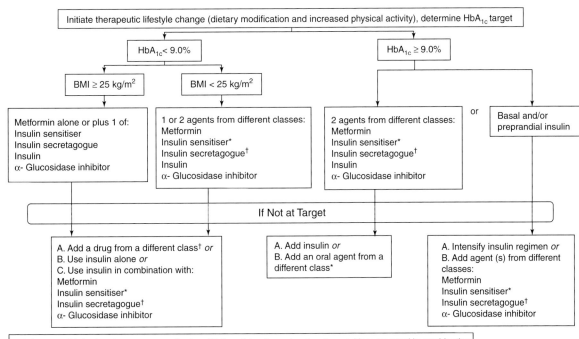

Figure 10.1 Management of hyperglycaemia in type 2 diabetes.
Source: Adapted with permission from Ref. 9.
Further treatment algorithms for initiation and adjustment of insulin regimens and metabolic management of type 2 diabetes can be found in Ref. 8.

Table 10.3 Expected decrease in HbA_{1c} with antihyperglycaemic therapy

Agent/class of agent	Expected decrease in HbA_{1c} (%)
Metformin	1.1–3.0
Insulin secretagogues	
Sulphonylureas	0.9–2.5
Meglitinides	0.5–1.5*
Insulin sensitisers (thiazolidinediones)	1.5–1.6
α-Glucosidase inhibitor (acarbose)	0.6–1.3
Dipeptidyl-peptidase 4 inhibitors	0.8
Exenatide	0.8–0.9
Insulin	Depends on regimen

For comparison, exercise may reduce HbA_{1c} by 1–2% and weight loss by even more.
*0.5–1.0 for nateglinide, 1.0–1.5 for repaglinide.
Source: Refs. 8 and 9.

Table 10.4 Key contraindications to the use of antihyperglycaemic drugs

Condition	Contraindicated agents
Renal impairment	Metformin Sulphonylureas Exenatide
Hepatic disease	Metformin Thiazolidinediones
Cardiac failure	Metformin Thiazolidinediones
Some forms of intestinal disease	α-Glucosidase inhibitors
Any condition likely to be associated with tissue hypoxia and lactic acidosis (e.g. dehydration, acute myocardial infarction, sepsis, alcoholism)	Metformin

for intensification of therapy, and many patients who initially achieve adequate control with oral antihyperglycaemic agents eventually require insulin.

Insulin may be used alone or in combination with oral antihyperglycaemic agents in a number of patient groups (Figure 10.1). Addition of insulin to the therapeutic regimen is usually recommended for patients who have failed to achieve target plasma glucose levels in response to the combination of lifestyle changes and treatment with oral hypoglycaemic agents and for patients with marked hyperglycaemia ($HbA_{1c} > 9.0\%$).[15]

One successful regimen (see Box 10.3) involves the addition of a single bedtime injection of intermediate-acting insulin, long-acting insulin or extended long-acting insulin analogue (insulin glargine or detemir) to oral antihyperglycaemic agents.

Table 10.5 Main adverse events associated with antihyperglycaemic agents

Agent/class of agent	Side effect
Metformin	Gastrointestinal intolerance
Sulphonylureas	Hypoglycaemia Weight gain
Meglitinides	Hypoglycaemia Weight gain
α-Glucosidase inhibitors	Gastrointestinal intolerance
Thiazolidinediones	Weight gain Fluid retention and oedema Congestive heart failure in patients at risk
Dipeptidyl-peptidase 4 inhibitors	No clinically significant side effects
Insulin	Hypoglycaemia Weight gain Fluid retention and oedema (rare)

This type of therapeutic regimen is suitable for patients with good secretory reserve of insulin. Another frequently used regimen involves twice daily administration of pre-mixed (fast-acting + intermediate-acting) insulin, although with the increasing prevalence of type 2 diabetes in the young there is also increased usage of multiple daily insulin injections (fast-acting mealtime insulin tid ± intermediate-acting insulin or extended long-acting insulin analogue at bedtime or bid). However, there is currently no compelling evidence of the superiority of one particular insulin type or regimen over another. The choice of insulin preparation and the frequency and timing of insulin injections will depend on the individual patient's circumstances and clinician preference, with the key outcome being achievement of glycaemic targets with minimal hypoglycaemia. The clinician is advised to develop experience in the use of one or two specific insulin regimens and to determine which inter-meal period (e.g. breakfast to lunch) is controlled by which component of the insulin regimen; patient self-testing data can then be used to adjust the dose of each component accordingly.

Box 10.3 Starting insulin in a patient with type 2 diabetes.

When?

- if glucose levels are unacceptably high for this patient, usually HbA$_{1c}$ > 7%
- if the patient is doing as well as they can or will with weight and exercise
- if the patient is on maximum (tolerated) metformin and sulphonylurea

1. Pre-warn the patient; this can usually be done many months in advance. Give a positive message
   - they will feel better
   - everyone finds it much easier than they expected

2. The patient needs to know how to test their own glucose at home with a meter. The Practice Nurse can teach them. Currently Accu-Chek Advantage meter and Medisense Optium are available on script. Lancets are not free, and are available from pharmacies (or Diabetes Auckland or Diabetes NZ via mail order).

3. Script Protaphane Penfill + needles (up to 100 subsidised) and give Novopen (available free from NovoNordisk); or Humulin N 3 mL for pen + needles, and give BD pen (available free from Eli Lilly).

4. Bring the patient in at the end of day to see you or the Practice Nurse. Tell the patient he/she will give first injection. Demonstrate dialling up 10 U and injecting into air. Get the patient to do it, then pull up their shirt / blouse, take a pinch of skin between thumb and forefinger, push needle vertically into top of raised skin, push plunger and withdraw.

5. If the patient is on bd metformin and sulphonylurea, stop their evening sulphonylurea from that day, and reduce metformin to bd if on tid.

6. The patient needs to check and record fasting glucose each morning for present.

7. Bring the patient back into surgery daily at much the same time until you/Practice Nurse and patient are happy that patient can continue unsupervised at home. Patients are usually confident after the initial visit and one or perhaps two more. Shift injection time at home to about 9 pm. Educate about hypos, though in practice they are highly unlikely.

8. The patient phones in fasting glucose readings, initially daily. You /Practice Nurse instruct to increase insulin dose, initially in 2 U increments every 2 days. Later, increase by 5 U if fasting glucose is not quickly decreasing. This works remarkably simply – often the initial dose and initial increases make no difference until fasting glucose starts to come down, then as insulin steadily goes up, glucose steadily comes down. Aim for a fasting glucose of about 6.

9. As fasting glucose decreases, ask the patient to check their glucose before lunch and before their evening meal, as the glucose will start to drop then. Reduce or stop sulphonylurea therapy. You should not need to reduce metformin – it is better to reduce insulin.

10. If the patient gets to 40 U insulin at 9 pm, switch to bd insulin, either the same insulin or a mixed short / intermediate.

Tim Kenealy Nov 06

Monitoring glucose control in patients receiving antihyperglycaemic therapy

Glycaemic control should be assessed using a combination of HbA_{1c} levels and patient self-monitoring of blood glucose. The latter is an important component of diabetes care and patients should be carefully educated in its use. When performed accurately, self-monitoring can be used to balance medication, nutritional intake and physical activity, and to prevent hypoglycaemia. Frequent blood glucose self-assessment is particularly important after initiation of insulin therapy and any change in insulin regimen to ensure that the patient is not at risk of hypoglycaemia and that blood glucose targets are reached.

Glycosylated haemoglobin (HbA_{1c}) reflects mean glycaemia over the preceding 2–3 months. This parameter should therefore be measured approximately every 3 months in patients whose blood glucose is inadequately controlled and in those patients whose therapeutic regimen has been changed. For patients who have stable glucose levels and who are meeting treatment goals, half-yearly assessment of HbA_{1c} is likely to be sufficient.

The risk of hypoglycaemia

Patients undergoing treatment with insulin and insulin secretagogues are at risk of hypoglycaemia and should be educated to recognise and prevent this adverse effect. For certain patient groups, such as children, those with hypoglycaemia unawareness, significant comorbidities, socially isolated patients, the elderly and those with limited life expectancy, the risk of hypoglycaemia may outweigh the benefits of tight glycaemic control; in such cases, a target HbA_{1c} level of $>7.0\%$ may be appropriate.

Conclusions

Diabetes is characterised by hyperglycaemia, and control of this metabolic derangement is a fundamental component of any therapeutic regimen to limit the microvascular and macrovascular complications of diabetes. Various oral antihyperglycaemic agents and insulins are available for treatment of type 2 diabetes, and these can be used alone or in combination, or in conjunction with insulin. The choice of therapeutic regimen is governed by clinical trial evidence, current and target HbA_{1c} levels, the patient's individual characteristics and physician preference. An HbA_{1c} target of $<7\%$ is currently recommended for most diabetic patients, and the aim should be to achieve this within 6 months of diagnosis. Most glucose-lowering therapies carry a risk of hypoglycaemia.

References

1. Rohlfing CL, Wiedmeyer H-M, Little RR, et al. Defining the relationship between plasma glucose and HbA_{1c}: Analysis of glucose profiles and HbA_{1c} in the Diabetes Control and Complications Trial. *Diabetes Care.* 2002; 25: 275–8.
2. Ohkubo Y, Kishikawa H, Araki E, et al. Intensive insulin therapy prevents the progression of diabetic microvascular complications in Japanese patients with non-insulin-dependent diabetes mellitus: A randomized prospective 6-year study. *Diabetes Res Clin Pract.* 1995; 28: 103–17.
3. Stratton IM, Adler AI, Neil HA, et al. Association of glycaemia with macrovascular and microvascular complications of type 2 diabetes (UKPDS 35): Prospective observational study. *BMJ.* 2000; 321 (7258): 405–12.
4. Diabetes Control and Complications Trial Research Group. The effect of intensive treatment of diabetes on the development and progression of long-term complications in insulin-dependent diabetes mellitus. *N Engl J Med.* 1993; 329: 977–86.
5. Nathan DM, Cleary PA, Backlund JY, et al. for the Diabetes Control and Complications Trial/Epidemiology of Diabetes Interventions and Complications (DCCT/EDIC) Study Research Group. Intensive diabetes treatment and cardiovascular disease in patients with type 1 diabetes. *N Engl J Med.* 2005; 353; 2643–53.
6. Turner RC, Millns H, Neil HA, et al. Risk factors for coronary artery disease in non-insulin dependent diabetes mellitus: United Kingdom Prospective Diabetes Study (UKPDS: 23). *BMJ.* 1998; 316 (7134): 823–8.
7. 2007 Clinical Practice Recommendations. Standards of Medical Care in Diabetes. *Diabetes Care.* 2007; 30 (Suppl 1): S3–103.
8. AACE Diabetes Mellitus Clinical Practice Guidelines Task Force. American Association of Clinical Endocrinologists medical guidelines for clinical practice for the management of diabetes mellitus. *Endocr Pract.* 2007 May–Jun; 13 (Suppl 1): 1–68.
9. Canadian Diabetes Association Clinical Practice Guidelines Expert Committee. *Can J Diabetes.* 2003; 27 (Suppl 2): S1–152.
10. Nathan DM, Buse JB, Davidson MB, Heine RJ, Holman RR, Sherwin R, Zinman B; Professional Practice Committee, American Diabetes Association; European Association for the Study of Diabetes. Management of hyperglycaemia in type 2 diabetes: a consensus algorithm for the initiation and adjustment of therapy. A consensus statement from the American Diabetes Association and the European Association for the Study of Diabetes. *Diabetologia.* 2006 Aug; 49(8): 1711–21.
11. Del Prato S, Felton AM, Munro N, et al. Global Partnership for Effective Diabetes Management. Improving glucose management: Ten steps to get more patients with type 2 diabetes to glycaemic control. *Int J Clin Pract.* 2005; 59: 1345–55.
12. ADVANCE Collaborative Group, Intensive blood glucose control and vascular outcomes in patients with type 2 diabetes. N Engl J Med. 2008; 358(24): 2560–72.
13. Action to Control Cardiovascular Risk in Diabetes Study Group, Effects of intensive glucose lowering in type 2 diabetes. N Engl J Med. 2008; 358(24): 2545–59.
14. UK Prospective Diabetes Study (UKPDS) Group. Effect of intensive blood-glucose control with metformin on complications in overweight patients with type 2 diabetes (UKPDS 34). *Lancet.* 1998; 352: 854–65.
15. UK Prospective Diabetes Study (UKPDS) Group. Intensive blood-glucose control with sulphonylureas or insulin compared with conventional treatment and risk of complications in patients with type 2 diabetes (UKPDS 33). *Lancet.* 1998; 352: 837–53.

11 Long-term management of cardiovascular disease

S.A. Brunton[1], A. Fitton[2] and A.G. Olsson[3]

[1]Cabarrus Family Medicine Residency, Charlotte, North Carolina, USA
[2]The Future Forum Secretariat, London, UK
[3]Faculty of Health Sciences, Linköping University, Sweden

Introduction

Clinical trials have established the benefits of lifestyle changes and pharmacotherapy in prevention of cardiovascular disease in patients with atherosclerotic disease, or at high risk of developing the disease. Most of these patients will require long-term management, comprising continual assessment and, if necessary, modification of the management strategy to achieve and maintain therapeutic goals. However, despite the availability of well-defined strategies for reducing cardiovascular risk, many patients are not offered adequate preventive care or lack the interest or motivation to undertake intensive risk-factor modification. Failure to address lifestyle issues such as obesity and smoking can prevent patients from achieving cardiovascular risk-reduction targets.[1] This is illustrated by the results of EUROASPIRE III survey, which showed that despite impressive increases in the use of cardiovascular medications including statins and all classes of antihypertensive therapies except calcium-channel blockers, blood pressure management has shown no improvement in the 12 years since the EUROASPIRE surveys started.[2–4] The lack of improvement in outcome is likely to be because smoking levels have remained the same, increasing in some groups, and body weight has dramatically increased in survey participants. Furthermore, the prevalence of diabetes has risen from 17% in the first survey to 28%.

Implementation of guideline recommendations requires an organised, coordinated approach, with well-defined healthcare team structures and roles. This article aims to provide practitioners with a guide to the long-term management of cardiovascular disease, including strategies to improve patient compliance. For further background the reader is referred to Ref. 5.

Cardiovascular Risk Management, Edited by R Hobbs and B Arroll
© 2009 Blackwell Publishing, ISBN: 9781405155755

The importance of follow-up

Patients at risk of cardiovascular disease should be followed up at regular intervals during treatment. The frequency of follow-up visits will be dictated by disease complexity, the level of symptom control and the degree of treatment compliance. Once treatment goals have been achieved, the follow-up interval may be extended to once a year. Follow-up visits provide the opportunity to ascertain whether treatment targets are being achieved, to reconsider alternative treatment options if necessary, to monitor patient compliance and to educate and motivate patients. Behaviour change research suggests that attendance at follow-up visits is the best predictor of achieving treatment goals.

Suboptimal treatment compliance

The benefits that might be gained from applying clinical guideline recommendations are often unrealised because a sizable proportion of patients fail to comply fully with their treatment programme.

Lifestyle changes are challenging for both the clinician and the patient. Behavioural counselling can help patients acquire the skills and motivation needed to alter their daily lifestyles; however, recent surveys suggest that the behavioural advice provided in routine clinical practice is often inadequate. In addition, many patients with cardiovascular disease require polytherapy, and these patients frequently show suboptimal daily compliance and low long-term persistence with their various treatment regimens. It is well established that compliance and long-term persistence with therapy tend to decline as the number of prescribed daily doses increases, and a similar relationship probably applies in the case of lifestyle changes.

Reasons for non-compliance

The reasons for non-compliance and lack of persistence with treatment are varied (Box 11.1). Compliance is influenced by

Box 11.1 Reasons for non-compliance with treatment

- Patient does not perceive physical harm from asymptomatic cardiovascular disease
- Incomplete or incorrect information/understanding of cardiovascular disease and its treatment
- Treatment-related side effects
- Complex dosing regimens
- Cost of treatment
- Poor cognitive abilities
- Low level of literacy
- Lack of family/social support

Box 11.2 Persistence-enhancing interventions for long-term cardiovascular disease management

- Involve the patient in treatment decisions and negotiate goals
- Simplify treatment regimens
- Provide the patient with clear instructions and information
- Encourage use of reminders for medication adherence
- Encourage the support of family and friends
- Monitor progress towards goals
- Schedule regular follow-up visits particularly for persons unable to achieve treatment goal
- Reinforce and reward compliance at each clinic visit
- Develop multicomponent strategies

the patient's level of literacy and understanding of his/her disease (a factor often overlooked by physicians), the nature of the recommended behavioural modification, the complexity of the treatment regimen and the ease with which the behavioural/treatment recommendations can be incorporated into the patient's daily routine. Compliance is also affected by the incentive vs therapeutic intent or goal and the ability to pay for care. It is difficult to predict a patient's likely degree of compliance with a given behavioural modification – compliance is not related to gender, age (although cognitive issues in the elderly may play a role) or ethnic or socioeconomic group. A patient may choose not to have the initial prescription filled, may successfully initiate therapy only to abandon it after a few weeks or months or may comply with only certain elements of a lifestyle or treatment regimen and thus fail to achieve optimal control. Research indicates that most patients do not successfully comply with prescribed behavioural or therapeutic interventions without outside assistance. Since there is no single cause of poor compliance, no one intervention is likely to improve compliance in all patients. Moreover, good initial compliance does not mean that the patient will persist with treatment.

Approaches for improving treatment compliance

There are several approaches that the physician can adopt to promote patient compliance (Box 11.2). Educating and motivating patients to understand the need for persistence with treatment is important in ensuring that the benefits of cardiovascular disease management, as demonstrated in clinical trials, are translated to the general population.[6] Also, simplification of the drug regimen can improve compliance, as most patients will require multiple therapies.[7]

Simplifying the treatment regimen

Recently, a novel approach to simplifying cardiovascular drug therapy – the polypill, which incorporates five low-dose drugs (three antihypertensives, aspirin and a statin) with or without folic acid into a single daily pill – has been proposed for prophylaxis of cardiovascular disease (Boxes 11.3 and 11.4).[8] It is suggested that this drug combination could be made widely available for primary prevention, without treating specific risk factors or individuals. However, the polypill strategy is still only theoretical, and there are important gaps in our knowledge about its likely benefits and risks. In addition to uncertainty about the cardiovascular benefits of routine use of folic acid, direct evidence of the effectiveness of simultaneous intervention against multiple cardiovascular risk factors is lacking. Furthermore, the cost-effectiveness of a non-targeted treatment approach (it is proposed that the polypill should be given to all adults over 55 years of age) is not known. However, the scale of the task of implementing cardiovascular disease prevention may necessitate novel simplistic strategies such as the polypill, and the effects of multiple combined medications on compliance should be explored.

Regardless of the chosen treatment approach, any intervention to improve adherence is effective only for as long as it is provided to the patient. Most successful interventions, especially for long-term drug therapy, rely upon multiple approaches.

Patient education

Patient education, if appropriately tailored to the patient's understanding and awareness of their disease, can have a positive impact on adherence with medication. Patients should understand that any prescribed medication will probably need to be continued indefinitely. However, patients' perception of their disease affects their motivation to persist with treatment – if the condition is largely asymptomatic, the patient is less likely to be persuaded of the need for continued treatment. Adherence with medication is related to the balance between a patient's belief about the necessity of treatment and their concerns about possible adverse effects. By improving patients' understanding of cardiovascular risk and the need for long-term treatment, and by addressing their apprehensions, physicians may influence treatment adherence.

Box 11.3 The polypill concept

Papers

A strategy to reduce cardiovascular disease by more than 80%

N J Wald, M R Law

Abstract

Objectives To determine the combination of drugs and vitamins, and their doses, for use in a single daily pill to achieve a large effect in preventing cardiovascular disease with minimal adverse effects. The strategy was to simultaneously reduce four cardiovascular risk factors (low density lipoprotein cholesterol, blood pressure, serum homocysteine, and platelet function) regardless of pretreatment levels.
Design We quantified the efficacy and adverse effects of the proposed formulation from published meta-analyses of randomised trials and cohort studies and a meta-analysis of 15 trials of low dose (50-125 mg/day) aspirin.
Outcome measures Proportional reduction in ischaemic heart disease (IHD) events and strokes; life years gained; and prevalence of adverse effects.
Results The formulation which met our objectives was: a statin (for example, atorvastatin (daily dose 10 mg) or simvastatin (40 mg)); three blood pressure lowering drugs (for example, a thiazide, a β blocker, and an angiotensin converting enzyme inhibitor), each at half standard dose; folic acid (0.8 mg); and aspirin (75 mg). We estimate that the combination (which we call the Polypill) reduces IHD events by 88% (95% confidence interval 84% to 91%) and stroke by 80% (71% to 87%). One third of people taking this pill from age 55 would benefit, gaining on average about 11 years of life free from an IHD event or stroke. Summing the adverse effects of the components observed in randomised trials shows that the Polypill would cause symptoms in 8-15% of people (depending on the precise formulation).
Conclusion The Polypill strategy could largely prevent heart attacks and stroke if taken by everyone aged 55 and older and everyone with existing cardiovascular disease. It would be acceptably safe and with widespread use would have a greater impact on the prevention of disease in the Western world than any other single intervention.

Introduction

Heart attacks, stroke, and other preventable cardiovascular diseases kill or seriously affect half the population of Britain. Western diet and lifestyle have increased the population levels of several of the causal "risk factors," and their combined effects have made the diseases common. Cardiovascular disease can be avoided or delayed, but the necessary changes to Western diet and lifestyle are not practicable in the short term. Randomised trials show that drugs to lower three risk factors—low density lipoprotein (LDL) cholesterol,[1] blood pressure,[2-6] and platelet function (with aspirin)[7 8]—reduce the incidence of ischaemic heart disease (IHD) events and stroke. Evidence that lowering serum homocysteine (with folic acid) reduces the risk of these diseases is largely observational but still compelling.[9 10]

Drug treatment to prevent IHD events and stroke has generally been limited to single risk factors, to targeting the minority of patients with values in the tail of the risk factor distribution, and to reducing the risk factors to "average" population values. This policy can achieve only modest reductions in disease.[11] A large preventive effect would require intervention in everyone at increased risk irrespective of the risk factor levels; intervention on several reversible causal risk factors together; and reducing these risk factors by as much as possible.[11]

We describe a strategy to prevent cardiovascular disease based on these three principles[12] and quantify the overall preventive effect. We show that a daily treatment, the Polypill, comprising six components, each lowering one of the above four risk factors, would prevent more than 80% of IHD events and strokes, with a low risk of adverse effects. This strategy would be suitable for people with known cardiovascular disease and for everyone over a specified age (say 55), without requiring risk factors to be measured.

Methods

We identified categories of drugs or vitamins used to modify LDL cholesterol, blood pressure, homocysteine, and platelet function. For LDL cholesterol, statins are the drugs of choice.[1 13 14] For lowering blood pressure, we considered all five main categories of drugs: thiazides, β blockers, angiotensin converting enzyme (ACE) inhibitors, angiotensin II receptor antagonists, and calcium channel blockers.[13] Serum homocysteine is most effectively reduced by folic acid; vitamins B-6 and B-12 have relatively small effects.[15] Aspirin is the most widely used and least expensive antiplatelet agent.

The choices of statin and of the categories and doses of blood pressure lowering drugs were

Editorial by Rodgers

Department of Environmental and Preventive Medicine, Wolfson Institute of Preventive Medicine, Barts and the London, Queen Mary's School of Medicine and Dentistry, University of London, London EC1M 6BQ
N J Wald
professor
M R Law
professor

Correspondence to:
N J Wald
n.j.wald@qmul.ac.uk

bmj.com 2003;326:1419

Further tables appear on bmj.com

Source: Reproduced with permission from Ref. 8.

Box 11.4 Components of the proposed polypill

- Low-dose statin (e.g. atorvastatin 10 mg or simvastatin 40 mg)
- Three half-dose antihypertensive drugs
- Thiazide and/or β blocker and/or ACE inhibitor
- Aspirin (75 mg)
- ± Folic acid (0.8 mg)

Patients are unlikely to remember all the information imparted during the initial consultation, so it is important to reiterate key points, supply written information where appropriate and provide adequate follow-up care. Information provided in the form of booklets, tapes, interactive computer programmes and paper-based charts may be helpful in improving short-term treatment adherence and health outcomes.[9]

Patient motivation

Building the patient's motivation requires careful assessment of their readiness to undertake and maintain changes to their lifestyles. The patient must learn new strategies to help them adopt and maintain a new behaviour, especially when daily routines are interrupted. Although these strategies may differ for different behavioural and therapeutic interventions, whether cessation of smoking, modification of diet, encouragement of physical exercise or self-administration of a new course of drug treatment, certain common skills are required, such as problem solving, self-monitoring, developing prompts and reminder systems, identifying potential relapses into old behaviours, enlisting social support, setting appropriate and realistic goals and rewarding achievement of new behaviours. Moreover, multiple skills are often necessary to enable patients to comply with new behaviours and maintain them over time or give up established unhealthy behaviours. Asking a patient to modify multiple lifestyle behaviours, especially if he/she is asymptomatic, presents a particular challenge that underscores the need for long-term motivation and multiple skill sets.[10] To this end, it may be appropriate to address the patient's understanding of his/her risk and risk behaviours. A personalised example of the consequences of cardiovascular disease may prove useful in persuading the patient of the benefits of behavioural/therapeutic intervention and the need for long-term compliance. For those patients who have already experienced a cardiovascular event, apprehension of disease recurrence provides a powerful motive for persistence with treatment, although denial can be a factor in continuing risky behaviours.

Patient self-reminding

Even when equipped with the necessary motivation and skills, patients have difficulty in complying with behavioural/therapeutic programmes. Two aspects of compliance must be considered: errors of omission – delayed and omitted doses – occur frequently during drug therapy, while errors of commission are common with dietary and other lifestyle programmes.

Patients need to incorporate self-reminders into their daily routines, and they need advice on how to adapt to changes in their schedules and environment. Travel and holidays, for example, can lead to delays or omissions in taking medications and dietary errors such as increased intake of high-fat and high-salt foods.

Support

Support provided by family, friends and physicians is important for all patients who are engaged in lifestyle changes or pharmacotherapy, particularly for those with impaired cognitive ability. Family members can help remind patients to take medications and attend appointments and encourage them in their lifestyle changes.

With continued education, motivation and support, it is hoped that compliance with therapy will become habitual. It has been observed that compliance rates are higher once patients have been compliant with treatment for more than a year. However, educating and motivating patients can take time and collaborative care by nurses, pharmacists and other healthcare professionals is vital to ensure success in managing patients.

Organisation and delivery of care

Cardiovascular disease management can be divided into two broad categories: (i) centralised, hospital-based and specialist-led care and (ii) decentralised, community-based and multidisciplinary care. Most patients with cardiovascular risk factors can be managed successfully within the primary care setting, although specialist advice may be required in some cases (Box 11.5).

The primary care team provides multidisciplinary, team-based care involving systems for patient monitoring and recall, as well as patient education and support in the self-management of their condition. In addition to the primary care physician, other healthcare professionals such as nurses, dieticians and pharmacists can facilitate patient management. They have a useful role to play in educating patients (e.g. explaining the rationale for dietary change and selecting appropriate foods) as well as promoting and monitoring lifestyle changes. Randomised controlled trials have demonstrated the value of nurse-run clinics in improving patients' perceptions of cardiovascular risk and the benefits of long-term compliance.

Organisational barriers to delivery of long-term care

Clinical organisation may also present barriers to the implementation of long-term cardiovascular risk-reduction programmes (Box 11.6).[11] Historically, cardiology services have focused on acute patient management rather than on cardiovascular prevention. In addition, poor communication and misunderstanding between physicians may delay or prevent the introduction of preventative measures; For example, the

Box 11.5 Considerations for referral to specialist care

- Patients who have failed drug therapy, and for whom secondary causes have been excluded and dietary/other lifestyle measures have been tried
- Patients in whom drug therapy is contraindicated or poorly tolerated
- Patients with comorbidities that the primary care physician is uncomfortable managing
- Patients who request referral to a specialist

Box 11.6 Barriers to implementation of cardiovascular risk-reduction programmes[11]

Physician

- Problem-based focus
- Feedback on prevention is negative or neutral
- Time constraints
- Lack of incentives, including reimbursement
- Lack of training
- Poor knowledge of benefits
- Perceived ineffectiveness
- Lack of skills
- Lack of specialist–generalist communication
- Lack of perceived legitimacy

Healthcare setting (hospitals, practices, etc.)

- Acute care priority
- Lack of resources and facilities
- Lack of systems for preventive services
- Time and economic constraints
- Poor communication between specialty and primary care providers
- Lack of policies and standards

Box 11.7 Physician and practice approaches to improve patient management

1. Consistent use of guidelines
2. Prompts to manage risk factors
3. Standardised treatment plans
4. Standardised referral procedures
5. Regular evaluation of performance on treatment
6. Develop good practice systems for patients to receive cardiovascular care
7. Remind patients of appointments and follow-up visits
8. Utilise collaborative care

care setting, have an important role to play in improving patients' understanding of cardiovascular risk management.

References

1. JSB2: Joint British Societies Guidelines on Prevention of Cardiovascular Disease in Clinical Practice. *Heart* 2005; 91 (Suppl 5): V1–V52.
2. EUROASPIRE II Study Group. Lifestyle and risk factor management and use of drug therapies in coronary patients from 15 countries. Principal results from EUROASPIRE II Euro Heart Survey Programme. *Eur Heart J.* 2001; 22: 554–72.
3. EUROASPIRE I and II Groups. Clinical reality of coronary prevention guidelines: A comparison of EUROASPIRE I and II in nine countries. *Lancet* 2001; 357: 995–1001.
4. Nainggolan L. EUROASPIRE uninspiring: Obesity and smoking wipe out any gains. *Heartwire*, 4 September 2007. Available at http://www.medscape.com/viewarticle/562377 (Accessed October 2007).
5. Preventive cardiology. The challenge of translating guidelines on cardiovascular disease prevention into clinical practice. *Eur Heart J.* 2004; 6 (Suppl J): J1–J59.
6. Pearson T, Kopin L. Bridging the treatment gap: Improving compliance with lipid-modifying agents and therapeutic lifestyle changes. *Prev Cardiol.* 2003; 6(4): 204–11.
7. Haynes RB, McDonald H, Garg AX, et al. Interventions for helping patients to follow prescriptions for medications. *Cochrane Library.* 2003; 4: 1–50.
8. Wald NJ, Law MR. A strategy to reduce cardiovascular disease by more than 80%. *BMJ.* 2003; 326 (7404): 1419.
9. Edwards A, Elwyn G, Mulley A. Explaining risks: Turning numerical data into meaningful pictures. *BMJ.* 2002; 324 (7341): 827–30.
10. Miller NH, Hill M, Kottke T, et al. The multilevel compliance challenge: Recommendations for a call to action. A statement for healthcare professionals. *Circulation* 1997; 95(4): 1085–90.
11. Pearson TA, McBride PE, Miller NH, et al. Task Force 8. Organization of preventive cardiology service. *J Am Coll Cardiol.* 1996; 27: 1039–47.

Further reading

1. Haynes RB, Ackloo E, Sahota N, McDonald HP, Yao X. Interventions for enhancing medication adherence. *Cochrane Database of Systematic Reviews.* 2008, Issue 2. Art. No.: CD000011. DOI: 10.1002/14651858. CD000011.pub3.

cardiologist may consider initiation of lipid-lowering therapy, the responsibility of the primary care physician, whereas the primary care physician may assume that such therapy would have been initiated by the cardiologist if it had been needed. However, specific interventions are available to improve long-term patient management (Box 11.7).

Conclusions

Successful long-term management of cardiovascular risk is important in reducing the burden of cardiovascular morbidity and mortality. However, despite the benefits of risk-factor management, many patients fail to reach guideline goals. Inadequate patient education, coupled with poor patient motivation and compliance, may be a major reason. Healthcare professionals, particularly those working within the primary

12 Managing cardiovascular risk in the future

B. Arroll[1], C.R. Elley[1], A. Fitton[2] and H. Lebovitz[3]

[1]University of Auckland, Auckland, New Zealand
[2]The Future Forum Secretariat, London, UK
[3]State University of New York Health Science Center, New York, NY, USA

Introduction

Atherosclerotic cardiovascular disease (predominantly ischaemic heart disease and ischaemic stroke) is the leading cause of mortality in 5 of the 6 World Health Organization (WHO) worldwide regions (the exception being Africa), and accounts for one-third of all global deaths.[1] Increasingly, the cardiovascular disease patterns currently seen in the economically developed world are becoming established in developing countries, which now account for nearly 80% of the global cardiovascular mortality and morbidity burden.[2] The unprecedented increase in recent years of modifiable cardiovascular risk factors such as hypertension, smoking, hyperlipidaemia and diabetes, which are the root causes of this global cardiovascular disease epidemic, can be largely attributed to improved life expectancy and the adverse lifestyle changes that accompany urbanisation and industrialisation (increased fat and total calorie intake, increased tobacco consumption and decreased physical activity).

Concept of total cardiovascular risk

The combined effects of individual cardiovascular risk factors determine the individual's overall (total) risk, and modest increases in multiple risk factors often have a greater impact on total cardiovascular risk than a large increase in a single risk factor. Accordingly, individuals who have multiple risk factors are more likely to experience a cardiovascular disease event than those with a single risk factor.

Treatment strategies have, until recently, encouraged healthcare providers to treat 'hypertension', 'hypercholesterolaemia' and 'hyperglycaemia' despite emerging evidence that there is a continuum of cardiovascular risk across the range of blood pressure, glucose and cholesterol values seen in the general population. These terms are likely to fall into disuse as the focus moves away from lowering blood pressure, glucose and cholesterol levels below arbitrarily determined thresholds and towards managing continuous distributions of interactive cardiovascular risk. The term commonly used for this interactive cardiovascular risk is 'absolute risk'.

Comprehensive cardiovascular risk assessment

An equation for assessing individuals' cardiovascular risk was developed from the Framingham cohort study.[3] The principle of assessing total cardiovascular risk using this equation was first introduced in New Zealand in 1993 for control of blood pressure,[4] and subsequent clinical US and European guidelines for the management of hypertension and dyslipidaemia acknowledge the concept of total risk assessment as the basis for initiating drug treatment.[5–9] In general, the benefits of therapeutic and lifestyle interventions on particular cardiovascular risk factors are governed more by the level of overall cardiovascular disease risk than by the relative risk associated with a single specific risk factor. Since these interventions produce the same proportional reduction in cardiovascular disease risk regardless of the absolute level of risk, treating individuals and populations at highest risk represents the most cost-effective preventive strategy. Primary practice, however, too often remains focused on treating isolated risk factors rather than addressing total cardiovascular risk. If cardiovascular disease prevention activities are to achieve maximum impact, a shift is required in favour of an integrated approach that focuses on control of total cardiovascular risk (i.e. multiple risk-factor intervention) at both the individual and the population levels.

Comprehensive cardiovascular risk management

There is substantial room for improving cardiovascular disease prevention in the primary care setting and for implementing

Cardiovascular Risk Management, Edited by R Hobbs and B Arroll
© 2009 Blackwell Publishing, ISBN: 9781405155755

best-practice guidelines. Given the availability of cost-effective, evidence-based interventions for addressing comprehensive cardiovascular risk, the challenge is to reduce cardiovascular burden through the integrated management of cardiovascular risk. To this end, a number of approaches have been proposed to increase the reach of interventions to those at risk, facilitate patient follow-up and promote better adherence with therapeutic and lifestyle interventions. Adherence to cardiovascular medications over time can be as low as 50–60% in some populations.[10,11] Effective interventions to improve adherence are needed and could impact substantially on cardiovascular outcomes. The future development in the area of cardiovascular risk management and pharmacotherapy lies less in the discovery of new medications or deciding on specific class-superiority (apart from superiority in cost-effectiveness and side effect profile, for example of thiazide diuretics over angiotensin converting enzyme (ACE) inhibitors and calcium channel blockers as first line blood pressure lowering in general)[12] than the improved reach and adherence with existing agents because of the far greater potential for health benefit.[13,14] Two innovations under development are the electronic decision support and the polypill.

Electronic decision support systems

The primary care sector is largely geared towards treating acute, time-limited illnesses. It often lacks the elaborate information systems necessary to systematically identify those at risk, offer appropriate management and support the extensive patient follow-up that is integral to total cardiovascular risk management. Developments in electronic medical record (EMR) systems are likely to transform the way medicine is practised at the point of care by providing the primary care physician with up-to-date clinical information and decision support. Technology will allow the patient's most recent clinical data (obtained through an interface with an EMR) to be applied to computer-interpretable disease management guidelines, and provide the physician, on-line, with a detailed, best-evidence-based treatment plan that is locally relevant, patient-orientated and practice-focused.

This scenario-based decision support technology has been deployed for some time in the United States, Australia and in other countries where EMR systems are more widely used.[15] In New Zealand, for example, the PREDICT system – a web-based clinical decision support system – has been developed for individual patient cardiovascular disease risk management in primary care. PREDICT estimates the cardiovascular disease risk and likely treatment benefit and provides immediate evidence-based treatment recommendations. PREDICT uses information stored in practice computers, such as age, gender, recent blood pressure recordings and lipid tests, and thus minimises the input of information provided by the clinician. In addition to clinician advice, it provides hard copy information for patients.

The cardiovascular risk information is stored with an encrypted identifier through the internet enabling research with this anonymous data such as revalidating risk equations and linking to cardiovascular disease event data from hospitals. Improved cardiovascular health outcomes still need to be demonstrated using this technology.[16]

Combination pharmacotherapy

One proposal for improving cardiovascular risk factor control involves the provision of a polypill, for example, combining a statin, antihypertensive agents (a β-blocker and/or a diuretic and/or an ACE inhibitor) at half doses and aspirin (75 mg) to all adults over 55 years and to adults of all ages with diabetes or cardiovascular disease, regardless of risk factors. It is estimated that such a strategy, allowing simultaneous intervention on multiple potentially causal cardiovascular risk factors (lipids, blood pressure and platelet aggregation) in a broad swathe of the population-at-risk, could substantially reduce the incidence of ischaemic cardiovascular and cerebrovascular diseases.[17,18] Opposition to this standardised 'one-pill-for-all' approach to primary prevention centres on the fact that it does not necessarily control risk factors on an individual basis, and that higher-risk patients will remain under-treated. However, the polypill strategy is still only theoretical, and direct evidence of the effectiveness of simultaneous intervention against multiple cardiovascular risk factors is needed.

Interventions for reducing obesity

Weight loss, particularly in those at risk with metabolic syndrome, pre-diabetes or diabetes, can be successful using behaviourally based lifestyle interventions alone (such as dietary or physical interventions), or in combination with existing or emerging anti-obesity agents, or surgical interventions such as lap banding.

Counselling on physical activity

Primary health care is an ideal setting to identify sedentary individuals and deliver advice on physical activity, since more than 80% of adults visit their family physician at least once per year. Research from New Zealand indicates that clinic-based counselling (using the Green prescription) on the benefits of exercise, coupled with ongoing telephone support from exercise specialists, can result in sustained improvements in patients' physical activity and sense of well-being, as well as blood pressure reductions, particularly in those under 65 years.[19] If implemented on a wide scale, such a strategy could produce major health benefits for sedentary individuals.

Much of the future clinical research in cardiovascular management will need to focus on encouraging individuals to make greater lifestyle changes in terms of diet and exercise. Lifestyle coaches (personal trainers) may need to be employed in primary care settings to achieve such changes.

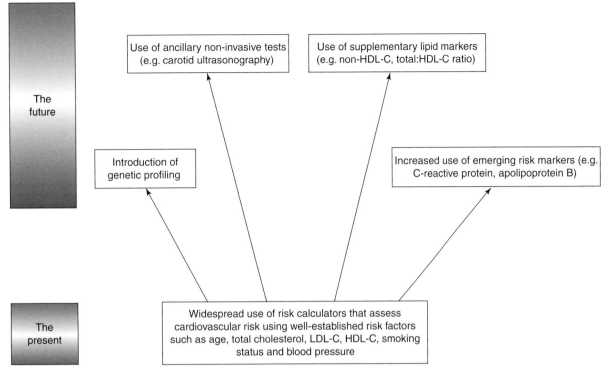

Figure 12.1 Current and future cardiovascular risk assessment.

Emerging risk markers

It is currently recommended that cardiovascular risk should be quantified using a risk calculator that incorporates well-recognised risk factors such as cholesterol level, blood pressure and smoking status (see Chapter 3) (Figure 12.1). In addition, there is a growing number of 'emerging risk markers' – notably C-reactive protein and apolipoprotein B – which may in future be more widely used in cardiovascular risk estimation.[20] Other risk markers are shown in Table 12.1. However, it is unlikely that addition of further markers will increase the precision markedly, and may impede every-day primary care use. Thus, existing risk charts using the most common risk factors are likely to maximise the use of the tool (e.g. Framingham or UKPDS equations). Additional markers may be more useful in subgroups or specialised settings. However, some improvements could be made in the actual equations for subgroups, such as those from different ethnic groups or those with co-morbidities, or pre-existing cardiovascular disease.[21,22] Work is underway in both of these areas.

Non-invasive techniques (e.g. carotid ultrasonography) as well as newer radiological investigations (e.g. CT angiography and CT calcium scoring) may also be helpful in estimating cardiovascular risk in some settings, whereas less well-established techniques such as genetic profiling may form a part of more specialised risk assessment in the future. Genetic profiling would allow at-risk individuals to be identified on the basis of genetic polymorphisms (e.g. cholesteryl ester transfer protein, apolipoprotein B) known to be associated with increased cardiovascular risk (Figure 12.1).[23] However, on a population basis the health benefit achieved from these advances is likely to be small compared with more effective delivery of existing strategies.

Table 12.1 Markers of cardiovascular risk

- C-reactive protein (CRP)
- Apolipoprotein B (or B:A ratio)
- Tissue factor
- Von Willebrand factor
- Flow-mediated dilatation (FMD)
- Vascular endothelial growth factor (VEGF)
- Homocysteine
- Plasminogen activator inhibitor (PAI-1)
- Oxidative factors:
  - isoprostane
  - xanthene oxidase
- Uric acid
- Matrix metalloproteinases (MMP) and their inhibitors (TIMP)
- B-type natriuretic peptide (BNP)
- Plasminogen activator inhibitor-1 (PAI-1)

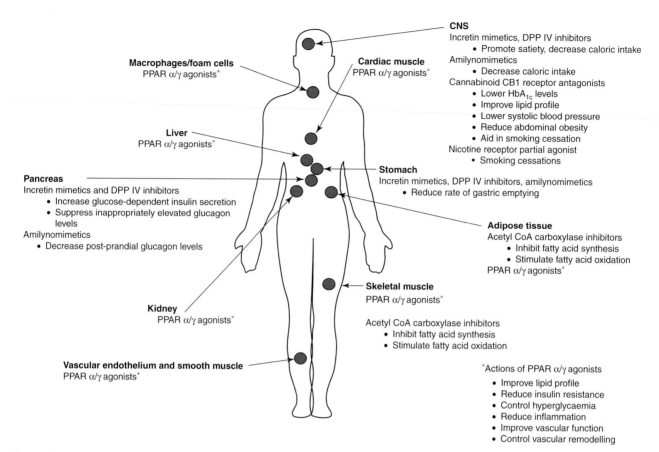

Figure 12.2 Agents for use in patients with type 2 diabetes or the metabolic syndrome.

Future drugs and strategies for cardiovascular risk reduction

Numerous pharmacological agents are currently being developed for use in cardiovascular risk reduction strategies. These include agents that increase HDL-cholesterol, agents that improve plasma lipid profiles, agents that lower blood pressure more effectively, agents that improve glycaemic control and gene therapy (Figure 12.2) (Table 12.2). In addition, gene therapy is being advocated as a potential adjunct or alternative to pharmacological therapy for patients with cardiovascular disease. In this technique, nucleic acid is transferred to the cells of the recipient with the aim of replacing the function of a defective gene, augmenting the synthesis of therapeutic proteins or blocking the expression of particular genes. Moreover, in the future, knowledge of a patient's genetic profile may allow pharmacological therapy to be tailored to his/her genome in some cases.[24,25]

Better drugs and greater adherence in taking blood pressure, lipid-lowering and hypoglycaemic medication will be needed if higher levels of control of cardiovascular risk factors are to be obtained. Systems for managing cardiovascular disease will need to be developed and implemented in primary care.[26]

Conclusions

Systematic cardiovascular risk assessment and management, delivered by general practitioners at an individual or a population level using electronic medical records and electronic decision support systems, coupled with innovative approaches to lifestyle changes and pharmaceutical intervention delivery and improved adherence, offers scope for enormous health gains in the primary care setting. This type of strategy, based on consideration of total cardiovascular risk and targeted at high-risk patients with good chronic care management systems in place, is likely to prove more effective, both clinically and economically, than the current opportunistic approach of treating individual cardiovascular risk factors.

Table 12.2 New and potential future therapies for cardiovascular risk reduction

Agents that increase HDL-cholesterol levels
- Lecithin:cholesterol acyltransferase (LCAT) inhibitors
- Gemcabene
- Nuclear receptor modulators (e.g. GW3965)
- Lipoprotein lipase activators (e.g. NO-1886)

Agents that lower plasma cholesterol levels
- Ileal apical sodium/bile acid cotransporter (IBAT) inhibitors (e.g. 264W94, S-8921)
- Sterol regulatory element binding protein cleavage-activating protein (SREBP) ligands
- Microsomal triglyceride transfer protein (MTP) inhibitors
- Squalene synthase inhibitors (e.g. TAK-475)
- Phytostanols (e.g. FM-VP4)

Agents that lower blood pressure
- Selective aldosterone blockers (e.g. epleronone)

Anti-obesity agents
- Cannabinoid CB1 receptor antagonists (e.g. rimonabant)

Agents that improve glycaemic control
- Incretin mimetics (e.g. exenatide)
- Dipeptidyl peptidase IV (DPP IV) inhibitors (e.g. vildagliptin)
- Amylinomimetics (e.g. pramlintide)
- Peroxisome proliferators activated receptor (PPAR) α/γ agonists

Agents that improve metabolic syndrome components
- Acetyl CoA carboxylase inhibitors
- Cannabinoid CB1 receptor antagonists (e.g. rimonabant)
- Peroxisome proliferators activated receptor (PPAR) α/γ agonists

Gene therapy

References

1. WHO report. Risks to Health 2002. Geneva, Switzerland: WHO, 2002.
2. Mathers CD, Lopez A, Stein C, et al. Deaths and disease burden by cause: Global burden of disease estimates for 2001 by World Bank Country Groups. In Disease Control Priorities Project Working Paper 18. 2001. National Institutes of Health, Bethesda, MD.
3. Anderson JL, Carlquist JF, Horne BD, et al. Cardiovascular pharmacogenomics: Current status, future prospects. *J Cardiovasc Pharmacol Ther*. 2003; 8: 71–83.
4. Jackson R, Barham P, Maling T, et al. The management of raised blood pressure in New Zealand. *BMJ*. 1993; 307: 107–10.
5. Third report of the National Cholesterol Education Program (NCEP) expert panel on detection, evaluation, and treatment of high blood cholesterol in adults (Adult Treatment Panel III) (2001). Expert Panel on Detection, Evaluation, and Treatment of High Blood Cholesterol in Adults. *JAMA*. 2001; 285:2486–97.
6. Grundy SM, Cleeman JI, Bairey CN, et al. 2004 update – Implications of Recent Clinical Trials for the National Cholesterol Education Program Adult Treatment Panel III Guidelines. *Circulation*. 2004; 110:227–39.
7. 2006 Clinical Practice Recommendations. Standards of Medical Care in Diabetes–2006. *Diabetes Care*. 2006; 29 (Suppl 1): S4–42.
8. Graham I, Atar AE, Borch-Johsen K, et al. European guidelines on cardiovascular disease prevention in clinical practice. *Eur J Cardiovasc Prev Rehabil*. 2007; 14 (Suppl 2): S1–113.
9. Rydén L, Standl E, Bartnik M, et al. Guidelines on diabetes, pre-diabetes, and cardiovascular diseases: Executive summary. *Eur Heart J*. 2007; 28: 88–136.
10. La Rosa JH, La Rosa JC. Enhancing drug compliance in lipid-lowering treatment. *Arch Fam Med*. 2000; 9: 1169–75.
11. Kulkarni SP, Alexander KP, Lytle B, et al. Long-term adherence with cardiovascular drug regimens. *Am Heart J*. 2006; 151 (1): 185–91.
12. ALLHAT Officers and Coordinators for the ALLHAT Collaborative Research Group. Major outcomes in high-risk hypertensive patients randomized to angiotensin-converting enzyme inhibitor or calcium channel blocker vs diuretic: The Antihypertensive and Lipid-Lowering Treatment to Prevent Heart Attack Trial (ALLHAT). *JAMA*. 2002; 288 (23): 2981–97.
13. Kravitz R. (2005). Doing things better vs doing better things. *Ann Fam Med*. 2005; 3 (6): 483–5.
14. Woolf S, Johnson R. The break-even point: When medical advances are less important than improving the fidelity with which they are delivered. *Ann Fam Med*. 2005; 3 (6): 545–52.
15. Beilby JJ, Duszynski AJ, Wilson A, et al. Electronic decision support systems at point of care: Trusting the *deus ex machina*. *Med J Aust*. 2005; 183: 99–100.
16. Garg A, Adhikari N, McDonald H, et al. Effects of computerized clinical decision support systems on practitioner performance and patient outcomes: A systematic review. *JAMA*. 2005; 293 (10): 1223–38.
17. Wald NJ, Law MR. A strategy to reduce cardiovascular disease by more than 80%. *BMJ*. 2003; 326: 1419.
18. Combination Pharmacotherapy and Public Health Research Working Group. Combination pharmacotherapy for cardiovascular disease. *Ann Intern Med*. 2005; 143: 593–9.
19. Elley CR, Kerse N, Arroll B, et al. Effectiveness of counseling patients on physical activity in general practice: Cluster randomized controlled trial. *BMJ*. 2003; 326: 793–9.
20. Ridker PM, Rifai N, Cook NR, et al. Non-HDL cholesterol, apolipoproteins A-I and B100, standard lipid measures, lipid ratios, and CRP as risk factors for cardiovascular disease in women. *JAMA*. 2005; 294: 326–33.
21. D'Agostino RS, Grundy S Sullivan LM, et al. Validation of the Framingham coronary heart disease prediction scores: Results of a multiple ethnic groups investigation. *JAMA*. 2001; 286 (2): 180–7.
22. D'Agostino RB, Russell MW, Huse DM, et al. Primary and subsequent coronary risk appraisal: New results from the Framingham study. *Am Heart J*. 2000; 139 (2 Pt 1): 272–81.
23. Gibbons GH, Liew CC, Goodarzi MO, et al. Genetic markers: Progress and potential for cardiovascular disease. *Circulation*. 2004; 109 (25 Suppl 1): IV47–58.
24. Day INM, Wilson DI. Science, medicine, and the future: Genetics and cardiovascular risk. *BMJ*. 2001; 323: 1409–12.
25. Anderson KM, Odell PM, Wilson PWF, et al. Cardiovascular disease risk profiles. *Am Heart J*. 1990; 121 (1 Pt 2): 293–8.
26. Wagner EH, Groves T. Care for chronic diseases. *BMJ*. 2002; 325: 913–4.

Appendix

Competing interests

FDR. Hobbs has received intermittent research funding, sponsorship or lecture fees from a variety of pharmaceutical companies that market products licensed for cardiovascular disease treatment or risk reduction, including AstraZeneca. Editorial support was provided by E Washbrook of The Future Forum Secretariat, London, UK, which is sponsored by an unrestricted grant from AstraZeneca.

L. Erhardt is a speaker and advisor for AstraZeneca, MSD and Pfizer. S Wells has a National Heart Foundation of New Zealand Research Fellowship. Editorial support was provided by E Washbrook of The Future Forum Secretariat, London, UK, which is sponsored by an unrestricted grant from AstraZeneca.

Editorial support was provided by E. Washbrook of The Future Forum Secretariat, London, UK, which is sponsored by an unrestricted grant from AstraZeneca.

J.I. Stewart and A. Tonkin are members of the Future Forum. A. Tonkin has received support from AstraZeneca, Bristol-Myers Squibb, Merck Sharp and Dohme, Pfizer and Sankyo Laboratories. J.I. Stewart has been reimbursed for advisory roles by the following companies: AstraZeneca, Oryx, McNeil and Fournier; and for education development or facilitation by: AstraZeneca, Lilly and Aventis Editorial support was provided by E. Washbrook of The Future Forum Secretariat, London, UK, which is funded by an unrestricted grant from AstraZeneca.

D. Duhot and C. Packard are members of the Future Forum. D. Duhot has received honoraria from AstraZeneca, Pfizer and the French Society of General Medicine (SFMG), and also has a partnership with Sanofi-Aventis. C. Packard has received research/honorarium from AstraZeneca, GlaxoSmithkline, MSD, Pfizer, Organon, Schering Plough and Unilever. Editorial support was provided by E. McGregor of the Future Forum Secretariat, which is supported by an unrestricted grant from AstraZeneca.

J. Mendive is a member of the Future Forum. Editorial support was provided by E. McGregor of the Future Forum Secretariat. The Future Forum is supported by an unrestricted grant fromAstraZeneca.

B. Arroll has received travel funds from the Future Forum, which is an educational foundation sponsored by AstraZeneca. He is also on the advisory board for the Pharmac educational seminars. Pharmac is the Government funded pharmaceutical purchasing agency in New Zealand. S. Mann is a member of the Cardiovascular Subcommittee giving medical advice to PHARMAC, the New Zealand Government's drug purchasing agency. He has served on advisory boards to AstraZeneca and Merck, Sharp and Dohme and has conducted educational sessions sponsored by these companies and by Pfizer. Editorial support was provided by A. Fitton and E. Washbrook of the Future Forum Secretariat. The Future Forum is supported by an unrestricted grant from AstraZeneca.

Dr. Lawrence Leiter and Dr. Tim Kenealy are members of the Future Forum. Editorial Support for this article was provided by A. Fitton of the Future Forum secretariat. The Future Forum is supported by an unrestricted grant from AstraZeneca.

S.A. Brunton and A.G. Olsson are members of the Future Forum. S.A. Brunton has acted As a consultant for, and received financial support from, AstraZeneca and Novo Nordisk. Editorial support for this article was provided by A. Fitton of the Future Forum Secretariat. The Future Forum is funded by an unrestricted grant from AstraZeneca.

B. Arroll and H. Lebovitz are members of the Future Forum. B. Arroll is on the advisory Board for the Pharmac educational seminars. Pharmac is the Government funded Pharmaceutical purchasing agency in New Zealand. Editorial support was provided by A. Fitton of the Future Forum Secretariat, which is funded by an unrestricted grant from AstraZeneca.

Index